Freud's Principal Case Studies Revisited

Freud's Principal Case Studies Revisited explores Freud's six principal case studies studies – Dora, Little Hans, Schreber, the Wolf Man, the Rat Man and the Young Homosexual Girl – through the lens of contemporary psychoanalytic practice.

Thirteen leading Freudian-Lacanian psychoanalysts reassess these cases in light of their significance to psychoanalytic theory and practice and consider their relevance in the twenty-first century. With new case material, theory, and analysis, the cases are critically re-invigorated and restored to a privileged place within psychoanalysis. Each of the cases is approached via a pairing of two psychoanalysts who engage with the clinical material, as well as with each other, in addressing their contributions to an assembled audience of clinicians, trainees and scholars.

This book will be of great interest to psychoanalysts in practice and in training as well as psychologists, psychotherapists and psychiatrists. It will also be relevant for academics and students of psychoanalytic studies, philosophy, critical and cultural theory, social studies, critical psychology, gender and sexuality studies and queer theory.

Helena Texier is a psychoanalyst in private practice. She was longtime editor of *THE LETTER: Lacanian Perspectives on Psychoanalysis*. She has been involved in psychoanalytic training and has been Chair of the Association for Psychoanalysis and Psychotherapy in Ireland (APPI). She is a director of the Freud Lacan institute (FLi), Dublin.

Eve Watson is involved in psychoanalytic practice, training, and research in Dublin, Ireland. Her co-edited books include *Critical Essays on the Drive: Lacanian Theory and Practice* (Routledge) and *Clinical Encounters in Sexuality: Psychoanalytic Practice and Queer Theory*. She is the academic director of the Freud Lacan institute (FLi), Dublin.

The Freud Lacan institute Lectures series

Freud's Principal Case Studies Revisited
Freudian-Lacanian Psychoanalysts Reconsider the Legacy
Edited by Helena Texier and Eve Watson

Freud's Principal Case Studies Revisited

Freudian-Lacanian Psychoanalysts
Reconsider the Legacy

Edited by Helena Texier
and Eve Watson

Routledge
Taylor & Francis Group

LONDON AND NEW YORK

Designed cover image: © Jean Texier

First published 2025
by Routledge
4 Park Square, Milton Park, Abingdon, Oxon OX14 4RN

and by Routledge
605 Third Avenue, New York, NY 10158

Routledge is an imprint of the Taylor & Francis Group, an informa business

British Library Cataloguing-in-Publication Data
A catalogue record for this book is available from the British Library

ISBN: 9781032663708 (hbk)
ISBN: 9781032663678 (pbk)
ISBN: 9781032663746 (ebk)

DOI: 10.4324/9781032663746

Typeset in Times New Roman
by KnowledgeWorks Global Ltd.

Contents

Abstracts   *x*
The Freud Lacan institute (FLi) Lectures Series Preface   *xvii*
Notes on the Editors   *xviii*
Notes on Contributors   *xix*
Acknowledgements   *xxii*

Introduction   1
HELENA TEXIER AND EVE WATSON

DORA
Fragment of an Analysis of a Case of Hysteria   7

1 **Hysteria, History, Her Story: Freud's Dora**   9
   OLGA COX CAMERON

2 **Return to Dora, Again and Again**   24
   JAMIESON WEBSTER

YOUNG HOMOSEXUAL WOMAN
Psychogenesis of a Case of Homosexuality
in a Woman   37

3 **Gender Anxiety as a Symptom of the Analyst**   39
   ANOUCHKA GROSE

4 **Girl, Interrupted**   50
   PATRICIA GHEROVICI

LITTLE HANS
Analysis of a Phobia in a Five-Year-Old Boy   75

5   Horses for Courses: Psychoanalysis and a Small Boy   77
    CAROL OWENS

6   Little Hans in Context   89
    KRISTEN HENNESSY

THE RAT MAN
Notes Upon a Case of Obsessional Neurosis   97

7   What We Can Still Learn from the Rat Man   99
    ASTRID GESSERT

8   Freud's Knight   109
    GUY LE GAUFEY

THE WOLF MAN
From the History of an Infantile Neurosis   119

9   The Wolf Man, Invented   121
    ANNIE G. ROGERS

10 The Wolf Man and Psychosis in the Post-Oedipal Era   134
    RIK LOOSE

JUDGE SCHREBER
Psychoanalytic Notes on an Autobiographical
Account of a Case of Paranoia   151

11 The Form and Matter of Hallucinations in Schreber's
    Message Phenomena   153
    LEON S. BRENNER

12 Judge Schreber: A Neuralgic Point of Social Tensions   167
    ROLF D. FLOR

TO CONCLUDE 181

Reading Freud's Case Studies Today 183
ANNE WORTHINGTON

Index *195*

Abstracts

DORA

1 Hysteria, History, Her Story: Freud's Dora

Olga Cox Cameron

The case history of Dora has been so often and so thoroughly looked at head on, that a different looking seemed called for. Accordingly, it has been approached in this chapter by way of both a backward and a forward lens. Historically, Freud's encounter with hysteria takes place at a very specific junction. Its social, sexual, medical and literary avatars are invoked to underline the constraints within which both Dora and Freud were bound. But also within these mostly superseded constraints, a very contemporary drama played a central role – that of *gaslighting*. The tension created by these competing narratives makes for what is arguably a great short story.

Keywords

Dora, Freud, gaslighting, hysteria, psychoanalysis, *sinthome*, symptom, transference

2 Return to Dora, Again and Again

Jamieson Webster

This chapter underlines the importance of Dora throughout Jacques Lacan's many seminars, looking at the way he returns to her case again and again to reinvigorate his thinking. Dora seems to play an outsized role at many crucial turning points in Lacan's life and thought. The author aims to track these shifting readings, along with highlighting their clinical importance. Finally, the presentation of two cases will show how the case of Dora still provides a relevant model for orienting in psychoanalytic practice over a century later.

Keywords

Dora, hysteria, hysteric's desire, Lacan, psychoanalysis, symptom

THE YOUNG HOMOSEXUAL WOMAN

3 Gender Anxiety as a Symptom of the Analyst

Anouchka Grose

Why do some psychoanalysts experience so much anxiety when working with gender nonconforming analysands? Is it really true that contemporary discourse around gender identity and sexual orientation closes down the possibility of asking questions in clinical practice? And how is normativity supported in some Freudian and Lacanian theory around queer and trans subjects? This chapter looks at Freud's famous case of female sexuality in order to open up questions around contemporary clinical practice. While the case was admirably radical in 1920, a century of change (in part, generated by psychoanalytic thinking) has revealed blind spots in the text. And, further into the twentieth and even twenty-first centuries, Lacanian analysts can present a forceful conservatism under the guise of the sovereign good of appearing to "question everything".

Keywords

homophobia, homosexual girl, psychoanalysis, psychoanalyst's anxiety, queer, symptom, transgender

4 Girl, Interrupted

Patricia Gherovici

This chapter explores the background and circumstances surrounding Freud's treatment of Margarethe Csonka Trautenegg (Gretl), pseudonym Sidonie Csillag, an 18-year-old homosexual girl who presented herself to analysis without a single symptom. Combining Freud's approach with Lacan's reading of the case, as well as some post-feminist critical readings of Diana Fuss and Judith Butler, the author explores the logic of the attempted suicide not as resulting from a frustrated desire to receive a child from her father, as Freud claims, but rather as resulting from being excluded from the family system of kinship. In suicidal ideation, death appears as a paradoxical life force, a force that allows for a re-birth. Thus, clinical work opens a path towards figuring out how to live with the death drive. Here death emerges not as the opposite of life but rather as a condition for life.

Keywords

acting out, homosexual girl, hysteria, *passage à l'acte*, psychoanalysis, sexuation, suicidal ideation, woman

LITTLE HANS

5 Horses for Courses: Psychoanalysis and a Small Boy
Carol Owens

This chapter sets out to re-examine the received claims of psychoanalytic scholarship on Freud's case of "Little Hans". The chapter begins by considering what Freud discovered in the case that allowed for it to be considered a paradigmatic exemplar of his concept of the castration complex, the nosological category of anxiety hysteria, and an aetiological theory of phobia. Next, the chapter turns to the analysis of the case executed by Lacan in his fourth seminar, *The Object Relation*, in particular, his rethinking of the Oedipus complex, and development of the concept of the paternal metaphor. Finally, Darian Leader's remarks from his re-examination of the case following the publication of the derestricted material are considered.

Keywords

anxiety hysteria, castration complex, Freud, Lacan, Little Hans, Oedipus complex, phobia, psychoanalysis

6 Little Hans in Context

Kristen Hennessy

This chapter explores the case of Herbert Graf. Arguing that the case of Little Hans is, in some ways, an instructive abstraction that teaches about childhood neurosis, the author looks at what can be learnt from considering the child, Herbert, in his singularity, beginning by reviewing the bits of Herbert's (rather difficult!) history that are known to the reader today. With an emphasis on the child's symptoms in the context of the complicated relationship between Herbert's parents and Freud, the chapter explores the ways in which the child's symptoms were an answer to what could not be spoken in the family system. Ultimately, the chapter reminds the analyst of the primary duty of those working with the young child in the clinic: the duty to allow the censored details of the family story to be told in words, rather than symptoms.

Keywords

child's anxiety, Little Hans, myth, neurosis, parental symptoms. phobia

THE RAT MAN

7 What We Can Still Learn from the Rat Man

Astrid Gessert

This chapter explores aspects of obsessional neurosis and its treatment from a Lacanian perspective, using Freud's case of the Rat Man as illustration. It highlights the obsessional's dilemma of dealing with desire, and typical strategies involved in this. Particular attention is paid to the passage that may lead obsessional subjects to seek help from an other when their defensive strategies fail. This may happen at a point when they are confronted with the possibility of an overwhelming enjoyment at the cost of losing themselves, and with the anxiety this evokes. With regard to the treatment, the author explores the kind of transference the analysand may develop, the position of the analyst, and what direction the treatment should take. Readers will find signposts to develop their understanding of the function of obsessional neurosis as well as guidance in respect of treatment.

Keywords

anxiety, Freud, *jouissance*, obsessional defences, obsessional neurosis, procrastination, Rat Man

8 Freud's Knight

Guy Le Gaufey

This chapter makes the case that when reading Freud's account of his treatment of the Rat Man, given in "Notes Upon a Case of Obsessional Neurosis", the reader must bear in mind the very particular contextual circumstances of the writing. Freud had been waiting for such a patient for almost ten years, this long interlude following the case of Mr. E whose 5-year-long treatment he had recounted to Wilhelm Fliess as it was ongoing. It must be added that even while Ernst Lanzer was still on the couch, Freud talked about this case many times, including during the first analytical congress in Salzburg, when he gave an exposition lasting five hours without an interval. Such a transference, from Freud to the Rat Man, can shed some light on the making of "obsessional neurosis" in the field of psychoanalysis.

Keywords

case presentation, Freud, obsessional neurosis, psychoanalytic practice, Rat Man, transference

THE WOLF MAN

9 The Wolf Man, Invented

Annie G. Rogers

This chapter revisits historic inventions of Sergei Pankejeff as the Wolf Man. Rogers begins with Freud's case, his diagnosis of obsessional neurosis grounded in the analysis of the famous dream of the white wolves, its origins in castration anxiety and, ultimately, in the primal scene. Despite the persuasiveness of Freud's arguments in the published case, the reader learns of his doubts and lingering questions through the fair copy revisions. Lacan, in presentations prior to his third seminar on psychosis, questions Freud's diagnosis. While Ruth Mack Brunswick followed Freud in her diagnosis and subsequent treatment of Mr. Pankejeff, she introduced an intervention so alarming that it precipitated hallucinations. Rogers extracts key concepts from Lacan's twenty-third seminar on psychosis to make yet another invention of the Wolf Man. She cites and questions each of the historic psychoanalytic inventions in the face of how little Sergei Pankejeff can say of his lived subjective experience in his memoirs (*The Wolf-Man by the Wolf-Man*), that it was a book written largely by psychoanalysts. Did he find a name and a place in psychoanalytic history by making himself as object of psychoanalysis? The reader may well wonder what analysts are inventing and reinventing as they continue to study and write about the Wolf Man.

Keywords

foreclosure, Freud, hysteria, Lacan, Mack Brunswick, obsessional neurosis, Pankejeff, psychoneuroses of defence, psychosis, Wolf Man

10 The Wolf Man and Psychosis in the Post-Oedipal Era

Rik Loose

This chapter re-examines Freud's complex and convoluted case of the Wolf Man with concepts and ideas developed by J.-A. Miller in cooperation with colleagues of the *Ecole de la Cause Freudienne*. The case is considered from a new perspective, a perspective that is based on Miller's proposed category of ordinary psychosis. Analytic experience and clinical data in our modern era – an era when psychoanalytically can be designated as post-Oedipal, an era in which the Name-of-the-Father has lost some (if not most) of its traction – have led to the proposal of the category of ordinary psychosis. The author's approach is to learn from the questions, confusions, complexities, and paradoxes of the Wolf Man case – a case that has been commented on many times over – in order to throw some (new) light on the changed landscape of madness in modern times, but also in order to indicate what some of the consequences are for the treatment of psychosis.

Keywords

Freud, Miller, ordinary psychosis, psychoanalysis, psychosis, Wolf Man

JUDGE SCHREBER

11 The Form and Matter of Hallucinations in Schreber's Message Phenomena

Leon S. Brenner

This chapter investigates the structural dynamics of hallucinations in psychotic experiences through the lens of Lacanian psychoanalysis. Drawing on Lacan's seminal work, "On a Question Prior to Any Possible Treatment of Psychosis" of 1958 and the autobiographical account of psychotic episodes by Daniel Paul Schreber, hallucinations are described not merely as perceptual distortions but as meaningful, subjective experiences that bear significance within the structural dynamics of psychosis. Central to the analysis is Lacan's concept of message phenomena, a type of hallucinatory experience characterised by incomplete or fragmented sentences that compel the subject into a process of meaning-making. These phenomena reveal existential questions about the subject's position in relation to the Other. The chapter concludes by arguing that the creative manipulation of language by psychotic subjects in the context of message phenomena serves as a stabilising force, allowing them to address the void left by psychotic foreclosure. This improvisational know-how with language enables subjects to actively recontextualise their experiences, leading to a unique form of narcissistic aesthetics that grants them a sense of certainty and personal meaning within their worlds.

Keywords

Freud, hallucination, Lacan, message phenomena, narcissistic aesthetics, psychoanalysis, psychotic experience, Schreber

12 Judge Schreber: A Neuralgic Point of Social Tensions

Rolf D. Flor

This chapter explores the psychiatric case of Daniel Paul Schreber, a German judge whose memoirs of his experiences with psychosis have influenced psychoanalytic thought, particularly through the work of Sigmund Freud and Jacques Lacan. The chapter delves into Schreber's autobiographical writings, which not only shed light on his personal struggle but also critique the medical and societal responses to his condition. The author examines how Schreber's narrative challenges neuro-reductionistic psychiatric models, advocating instead for a more dialogical approach in psychoanalysis that acknowledges the psychotic individual as an active participant in their treatment. Through this lens, the chapter offers insights into the potential of psychoanalysis to engage more deeply with the subjective experiences of individuals in extreme states, ultimately proposing a shift in how psychosis is understood and treated.

Keywords

delusion, extreme states, Freud, Lacan, neuro-reductionism, psychoanalysis, psychosis, Schreber, transference

TO CONCLUDE

Reading Freud's Case Studies Today

Anne Worthington

This chapter is a reading of Freud's collection of case studies of hysteria, 1893–1895, in response to claims that the knowledge he gleaned from his clinic has little relevance today and in response to concerns about the validity of the individual clinical case study as a methodology for the transmission of knowledge. These earliest case histories show how Freudian theory and practice have their origins in the individual encounters between analysand and analyst. In those encounters with suffering women who challenged both Freud and the very status of knowledge, he listens and learns. He learns about the effect of the relationship between "doctor and patient" – transference, about the trauma of sexuality and sexual difference, about the effects and functions of speech and language, about memory, about identification and so much more. The author introduces something of how Lacan took up Freud's radical ideas and with an illustration from events in 2011 in Le Roy, New York, suggests that Lacan's analysis of the structure of hysteria in its relentless interrogation of knowledge and of the Other's desire is of critical relevance today. She proposes that reading Freud's case studies today ensures the continuation of the challenge to accepted knowledge – as this volume illustrates.

Keywords

case studies as methodology, Freud, hysteria, Lacan, psychoanalysis, sexual difference, transference, trauma of sexuality

The Freud Lacan institute (FLi) Lectures Series Preface

Series Editors: Eve Watson and Helena Texier

Emerging from the lecture programmes and events organised by the Freud Lacan institute (FLi), this book constitutes Volume I of a two-volume collection. The work of the Freud Lacan institute is dedicated to the studies of Freud *and* Lacan in contemporary clinical contexts with cultural and literary specificities. The initial works will form part of a longer more extended series tied into future Freud Lacan institute activities and programmes, which are distinguished by drawing on *both* Freudian psychoanalysis and Lacanian psychoanalysis.

The first two volumes arise from two significant FLi events organised and held in Dublin. The first was a year-long online clinical programme of study dedicated to the examination of Freud's six major case studies in contemporary contexts which drew international speakers and attendees from around the world. The second event was a hybrid conference on James Joyce's writing, in the centenary year of the publication of *Ulysses*, which took place during November 2022 in Dublin. This drew speakers and attendees from all over the English-speaking psychoanalytic as well as Joyce studies world. Both events were characterised by the expression of interest for the papers to be published. The two events indicate a continued strong interest in both Freud's case studies and in the writing of James Joyce as highly pertinent to contemporary psychoanalytic thought and practice and socio-cultural studies.

The depth, richness, and contemporaneousness of the papers presented by leading practitioners and scholars in the field of Freudian Lacanian psychoanalysis and literary studies at these two innovative interactive and inter-disciplinary events made a compelling case for organising the accumulated material into publication as collections. It is envisaged that such important, relevant collections will strongly resonate with experienced practitioners in contemporary psychoanalysis, the burgeoning field of traineeship and psychoanalytic education, and scholars and students of English studies and literary studies.

FLi's future publications will continue along this rewarding vein, favouring a forward-looking and outward-facing ethos within which *instituting* replaces *institutionalising* knowledge.

The Editors

Helena Texier is a psychoanalyst in private practice in Dublin. She has taught psychoanalytic theory to postgraduates at the School of Psychotherapy in St. Vincent's University Hospital, Dublin (UCD), and at Trinity College Dublin (TCD). She was editor of *THE LETTER: Lacanian perspectives on psychoanalysis* from its inception in 1993 to 2003. She was Chair of the Association for Psychoanalysis and Psychotherapy in Ireland (APPI). She is a clinical fellow of the International Neuropsychoanalysis Association (NPSA). She is a director at the Freud Lacan institute (FLi).

Eve Watson is involved in psychoanalytic practice, training, education, and research in Dublin. She writes regularly for psychoanalytic journals and book collections. Her co-edited books are *Critical Essays on the Drive: Lacanian Theory and Practice* (Routledge, 2024) and *Clinical Encounters in Sexuality: Psychoanalytic Practice and Queer Theory* (2017, Punctum Books). She is the academic director of the Freud Lacan institute (FLi), Dublin, and from 2016–24 was the Editor of *Lacunae, the International Journal for Lacanian Psychoanalysis*. She was the 2022 Erik Erikson Scholar-in-Residence at the Austen Riggs Centre in Stockbridge, Massachusetts.

Contributors

Leon S. Brenner is a philosopher and psychoanalyst from Berlin. His work focuses on subjectivity theory and the understanding of the relationship between culture and psychopathology. His book, *The Autistic Subject: On the Threshold of Language*, was published with the Palgrave Lacan Series in 2020. Among his extensive international academic speaking and various publications, Brenner has made numerous appearances in interviews and video publications online. He is a founder of *Lacanian Affinities Berlin* and *Unconscious Berlin* and is currently a research fellow at the International Psychoanalytic University (IPU) Berlin and Ruhr-University Bochum.

Olga Cox Cameron is a psychoanalyst who has been in private practice in Dublin for the past 34 years. She lectured in psychoanalytic theory and also in psychoanalysis and literature at St. Vincent's University Hospital, Dublin and Trinity College Dublin from 1991–2013. She is the author of *Studying Seminar 6: Lacan's Seminar on Desire* (2021) and has published numerous articles on these topics in national and international journals. She is the founder of the annual Irish Psychoanalysis and Cinema Festival, now in its sixteenth year.

Rolf D. Flor is a psychoanalyst in private practice. He is Clinical Director for the Eliot Centre in Lynn, Massachusetts, where he oversees the training, education and supervision programmes. He has published in numerous journals and edited collections. He has taught at schools in the United States and Germany, most recently clinical practice at Boston College and Lacanian Theory at the Massachusetts Institute of Psychoanalysis.

Astrid Gessert is a psychoanalyst and a member of CFAR (Centre for Freudian Analysis and Research London, https://cfar.org.uk) and the College of Psychoanalysts – UK. She has worked for many years in the NHS, in private practice and as a supervisor. She is a regular contributor to the CFAR annual public lecture and training programme, and she lectures and facilitates at other psychoanalytic organisations' events. Her two books are edited collections, *Introductory Lectures on Lacan* (Routledge, 2014) and *Obsessional Neurosis: Lacanian Perspectives* (Routledge, 2018). She features in the well-known short series of videos about psychoanalysis made by the Freud Museum London.

Patricia Gherovici is a psychoanalyst, analytic supervisor, and recipient of the 2020 Sigourney Award for her clinical and scholarly work with Latinx and gender variant communities. She is a trustee at Pulsion: The International Institute of Psychoanalysis and Psychoanalytic Somatics, New York. Her single-authored books include *The Puerto Rican Syndrome* (2010) (Gradiva Award and Boyer Prize), *Please Select Your Gender: From the Invention of Hysteria to the Democratizing of Transgender* (2010) and *Transgender Psychoanalysis: A Lacanian Perspective on Sexual Difference* (2017). She co-authored with Chris Christian, *Psychoanalysis in the Barrios: Race, Class, and the Unconscious* (2018) (Gradiva Award and the American Board and Academy of Psychoanalysis Book Prize). She edited with Manya Steinkoler *Lacan on Madness: Yes You Can't* (2015), *Lacan, Psychoanalysis, and Comedy* (2016) and most recently *Psychoanalysis, Gender and Sexualities: From Feminism to Trans* (2023) (Gradiva Award for Best Edited Collection).

Anouchka Grose is a British-Australian Lacanian psychoanalyst and writer. She is a member of The Centre for Freudian Analysis and Research (CFAR), where she lectures. Her articles have been published in *The Guardian, The Independent*, and her short stories have appeared in *Granta Magazine* and *The Erotic Review*. Her books include an edited collection, *Hysteria Today* (Karnac: 2016) and *From Anxiety to Zoolander: Notes from Psychoanalysis* (Karnac, 2018).

Kristen Hennessy is a psychologist in private practice in rural Pennsylvania where she specialises in the treatment of children and adolescents in the "system". Her presentations include Lacanian clinical work with children and adolescents with histories of abuse, psychoanalysis and intellectual disability, traumatised masculinities, and the intersections of psychoanalysis and qualitative research. In addition to her work in the USA, she has experience developing and running psychoanalytically informed seminars for orphanage caregivers in Kenya. In 2022, she co-edited a collection with Chris Vanderwees, *Psychoanalysis, Politics, Oppression, and Resistance: Lacanian Perspectives* (Routledge, 2022).

Guy Le Gaufey was a member of *the École Freudienne de Paris* and co-founded the Lacanian journal *Littoral* and the *École lacanienne de psychanalyse*. He has written and published widely in French, English, and Spanish including his book, *Lacan and the Formulae of Sexuation: Exploring Logical Consistencies and Clinical Consequences* (Routledge, 2020). He has also translated books from English into French, including the work of Philip Larkin.

Rik Loose is a member of ICLO-NLS, APPI, the NLS (New Lacanian School) and the WAP (World Association of Psychoanalysis). He is former Head of Department of Psychoanalysis in Dublin Business School, School of Arts and former Senior Lecturer there and is the author of *The Subject of Addiction: Psychoanalysis and the Administration of Enjoyment* (Routledge, 2018) as well as numerous articles in the wider Lacanian field.

Carol Owens works in private practice in Dublin. Her book *Lacanian Psychoanalysis with Babies, Children, and Adolescents* (co-edited with Stephanie Farrelly Quinn) was published in 2017 (Karnac/Routledge) and nominated for the Gradiva Award. She has given seminars and talks on her work at national and international psychoanalytic events. Her most recent book is *Psychoanalysing Ambivalence with Freud and Lacan: On and Off the Couch* (with Stephanie Swales) published in 2020 (Routledge). She is the series editor for *Studying Lacan's Seminars* at Routledge.

Annie G. Rogers is Professor Emerita of Psychoanalysis and Clinical Psychology at Hampshire College and has a private practice in Amherst, Massachusetts. She is a supervising and teaching Analyst at the Lacanian School of Psychoanalysis in San Francisco. She is a printmaker and member of Zea Mays Printmaking in Florence, Massachusetts. Formerly a Fulbright Fellow at Trinity College, Dublin, Ireland; Radcliffe and Murray Fellow at Harvard University; Whiting Fellow at Hampshire College; and Erikson Scholar at Austen Riggs, Dr. Rogers is the author of *A Shining Affliction: A Story of Harm and Healing in Psychotherapy* (1995); *The Unsayable: The Hidden Language of Trauma* (2005); *Incandescent Alphabets: Psychosis and the Enigma of Language* (2016), and *After Words*: *A Novel* (2024).

Jean Texier designed the cover artwork to reflect the persons of the case studies as characters in a psychoanalytic story, taking his lead from the invented names by which they are more widely known. The cartoonish rendering serves to remind us that the real people behind the masks and the stories will remain somewhat mysterious to us, ultimately. Jean is an artist who has worked in the world of film animation for over 30 years. He is currently storyboarding film for Disney Studios. He is a freelance illustrator and painter.

Jamieson Webster is a psychoanalyst in private practice in New York City, part-time faculty at The New School for Social Research, and board member and faculty at Pulsion International Institute. She is the author most recently of *On Breathing* (Peninsula Press, UK; Catapult, US, 2025) and *Conversion Disorder: Listening to the Body in Psychoanalysis* (Columbia, 2018) and, with Simon Critchley, *Stay, Illusion! The Hamlet Doctrine* (Vintage Random House, 2013). She has written regularly for *Artforum*, *The New York Times*, *The New York Review of Books*, as well as many psychoanalytic publications.

Anne Worthington is a psychoanalyst, practising in South London. She is a member of the Centre for Freudian Analysis and Research (CFAR) and the Guild of Psychotherapists, contributing to their training programmes, and is a member of the College of Psychoanalysts – UK.

Acknowledgements

We would like to thank and applaud the courage and perspicacity of the 13 contributors to this collection who answered the challenge of re-visiting Freud's major case studies to critically reflect on their relevance more than a hundred years later and in the light of psychoanalytic practice today. This collection is, in effect, a fertilisation and elaboration of the work of these seminars in which a pair of presenters delved into one of Freud's major cases over the course of three seminars: Guy Le Gaufey and Astrid Gessert evaluated the Rat Man case; Rik Loose and Annie Rogers critically reflected on the Wolf Man; Kristen Hennessy and Carol Owens dedicated themselves to Little Hans; Leon Brenner and Rolf Flor delved into the Schreber case; Patricia Gherovici and Anouchka Grose re-evaluated the case of the young homosexual girl; Olga Cox Cameron and Jamieson Webster appraised the case of Dora; and Anne Worthington offered an incisive overview of Freud's casework and its relevance to the modern clinic. Readers will no doubt identify traces of the spoken aspect of the original presentations and notice the speaker-pairs engaging with and prompting each other to deeper analysis and elaboration. This is one of the many delights of this collection. The result – we suggest – is an exemplar, in its own right a template for clinical practice, for "re-visiting" a case, adding essential updates, moving with the changing times and presentations of suffering, to "hystericize" Freud's cases while refraining from the temptation to re-write them, as has become fashionable in some revisionist approaches.

We extend special thanks to Susannah Frearson, our publisher at Routledge, for her encouragement and support and without whom this collection would not be possible. We're grateful to Carol Owens, series advisor to the "Freud Lacan institute Lectures Series" in which this collection sits, for her unparalleled support. We offer our heartfelt appreciation to our co-founders and colleagues on the Board of the Freud Lacan institute, Martin Daly, Pauline O'Callaghan and Marie Walshe, and members, Therese Maguire and Micheli Romao for their collegiality and friendship. A special consideration is extended to Marie Walshe for her assistance in initiating this collection. We especially want to thank Jean Texier for taking time away from his storyboard desk to pick up on how the people behind Freud's case studies have been *character*-ised, and to devise and execute the cover artwork to give expression to that.

Finally, we'd like to acknowledge all the participants in the clinical programme of study 2021–2022 who made it one of the most spirited, exciting, and innovative programmes during an especially challenging time, and who inspired us in this project.

Introduction

Helena Texier and Eve Watson

Psychoanalysts – one foot in the nineteenth century and the other planted firmly in the twenty-first – have been talking and writing about Freud's cases continuously over a time-period spanning more than a hundred years. It would appear that we members of the psychoanalytic tribe are compelled to travel to a point of origin in the manner of wild salmon to their spawning grounds, or pilgrims to a hallowed place. The cases have been variously used; as means of introducing novices to the theory and practice of psychoanalysis, as a means of illustrating what distinguishes psychoanalysis from other forms of approach to psychological suffering, as a point of identification for psychoanalysts, as a point of divergence for psychoanalytic schools, as a starting point for renewal of the field, as an historical flag-bearer for a unique research methodology, and as a place-marker for perspective-taking in discussions of where the field now stands, no matter when the now. Whatever the era, every psychoanalytic generation goes back to go forward, and every generation's "return to Freud" has its own special character marked by its own contextual time. Ours – that of the Freud Lacan institute (FLi) – was no different. To use an Irish colloquialism, "the times that were in it" were exceptional. Our FLi return to Freud via the six major case studies constituted a psychoanalytic labour of love in a time of pandemic. This book brings the reader into contact with that collective work, involving participation of the international community of psychoanalysts, trainees, students, mental health professionals and the ordinarily curious. That very particular gathering, unique for its time, marked the beginning of what only a few years later we would consider commonplace – a virtual space for presentations where psychoanalysts from across the globe could come together to present their thoughts and formulations to an equally international audience, for discussion and critique. The feeling of broaching something new heightened the excitement and sense of importance of this project given over to a reconsideration of Freud's case studies, child of the impossible – when time appeared to stop and space collapse.

Freud famously proposed that psychoanalysis is no stranger to the impossible, being itself an impossible profession. The case study, as John Forrester puts it, is a pedagogical and institutional attempt to make up for this (2016, 65). As well as the six major case studies and the *Studies in Hysteria* (1893–1895), Freud's prolific writings are filled with rich and fascinating vignettes, cases, and clinical accounts

DOI: 10.4324/9781032663746-1

that deepen and enrich his theory expositions. They are, however, full of contradiction. On the one hand, they are richly descriptive and inspirationally creative, while, on the other, they lack any kind of uniformity. According to its title, Freud's longest case – Dora (1905) – is but "a fragment" of an analysis of a case of hysteria. The Rat Man (1909), although it is 104 pages long, is referred to as "Notes Upon a Case". The Wolf Man (1918) begins with Freud's startling disclaimer: "I have abstained from writing a complete history of his illness, of his treatment, and of his recovery, because I recognized that such a task was technically impractical and socially impermissible" (McGuire 1974, 8). In summary, Freud gave lengthy accounts of three patients, calling one a "fragment", a second "notes", and limiting the third to unravelling an infantile neurosis while telling us that it was "technically impractical", thus denying us the complete history of the case because such disclosure was socially unacceptable. There is also the case of Schreber (1911), whom Freud never met but analysed via his published memoir, and Little Hans (1909), who was the son of a colleague and whom Freud met only once during "the analysis". And there are the *Studies in Hysteria* which are important in their own right, none the least because they demonstrate Freud's approach to case presentation in the early stages of his development of psychoanalysis. This is an approach already informed by partiality, synopsis, problematics of revelation and concealment, questionable didactical usage, and the problem of transference.

As each of the contributors to this collection demonstrate in their analyses of Freud's major case studies and their relevance to psychoanalytic practice today, there is no such thing as just case content; there is the analysand's personal history, the way they attend to their story, the use of certain phrases and words, and there is always the relationship between the analyst and patient. There is also the question of the culture and episteme in which the case sits and how that influences it. The psychoanalyst, Ian Parker, notes that cases tend to be "saturated with elements of the psychoanalytic culture in which they were formulated" (2018, 29) and can end up being standardised, offering a single perspective of a "progress" of a case that meets with institutional criteria and not the meandering messy nature of treatment (p. 33). The astonishing beauty of Freud's cases derives from the way he presents to us the "meandering messy nature of treatment", filled as they are with gaps, elisions, and missteps in addition to the important elements that illustrate the main developments of the cases.

The problematics on one level arise from the "non-relation" between the analysand and analyst in so far as there is no "full" coincidence between them, no meeting of the minds, no unanimity of understanding possible; there are two subjects interacting via speech, coming from different and highly subjective positions who nonetheless find a way to address each other, in an attempt to make room for the new and the creative in the space proffered by this non-relation. John Forrester helpfully reminds us that psychoanalytic case presentation and writing are exemplary of a failure in so far as they end up symptomatizing what they are attempting to do; in their betrayal of the confidentiality of the setting, and by invoking a third party as partner or spectator they end up perversely betraying the founding condition of psychoanalysis. But he quite rightly asks, "Is there any human practice for which it is impossible to bear witness, and impossible to transmit, without betrayal?" (Forrester, 2016, 66). Especially when we factor in that, from a psychoanalytic standpoint, there are no human relations without transference and in order to transmit something of the work, this subjective transferential element shows that pure objectivity, strictly speaking, is impossible.

We can add to this Parker's assertion that something essential is lost in the transformation of one speech into another, in the re-presentation of the analysand's speech as a case presentation, in the synthetisation of hours and hours of discourse and affective flow into a clinical narrative (Parker, 2018, 6, 8) in which key points are indicated as insight or trauma or in a signifier, in seeking to capture the counterintuitive temporal logic of the clinic, when things shift, when the symptom begins to speak, when there is a cure, when the subject of the enunciation is enabled (p. 20). This occurs within a frame in which the analysand's truth is not transparent in direct speech but is found in error, omission, ellipses, and sometimes even in fiction and construction.

Yet it is impossible to imagine clinical formation, training, and ongoing practice without clinical casework which, for the most part, attempts to convey the unique experience of both the patient and analyst via either speech or writing. Are there forms of representation that can inscribe the very difficulties raised here, of the fact that in a psychoanalysis we work to facilitate the truth being spoken, even though the truth is, by definition, what slips away and is alienated within language; the truth of the subject can only be, as Lacan asserted, half-said and revealed in traces (1953, 215)?

The Structure of the Book

The 13 writers in this collection delve deep into the challenges of case "re-presentation" and do so by closely re-reading Freud's cases, unearthing new and surrounding material and re-contextualising the cases, and considering them in light of contemporary clinical practice. These writers re-think the cases and in so doing re-instil their value as essential supports to clinical practice today. But they do so with a caveat and one entirely in keeping with the times we live in – the cases require updating! This is in keeping with Lacan who repeatedly returned to Freud's cases throughout his life's work and re-evaluated them in support of a psychoanalytic practice attuned to what analysands say and not what analysts think. As Jamieson Webster puts it in Chapter 2, "Return to Dora, Again and Again", Lacan's attention to the cases "is a map for listening" and she reminds us that it took the hysteric, and importantly Dora, to "echo locate" the terrain of psychoanalytic treatment.

Carol Owens in Chapter 5, "Horses for Courses: Psychoanalysis and a Small Boy", invokes our positioning and "investment" when we read the cases and draws from her adolescent clinic in her analysis of Little Hans. Similarly, Olga Cox Cameron in Chapter 1, "Hysteria, History, Her Story: Freud's Dora", comments on how unconscious desire deflects the story being told and offers a perspicacious reading of Dora, highlighting the aspect of "fragment" and Lacan's "half-said". Kristen Hennessy in Chapter 6, "Little Hans in Context", asserts the practical importance of updating the theory for better clinical work in light of the modern clinic's challenges. She brings Little Hans to life with more clinical reality and detail, an approach each writer puts into effect in their re-reading of the cases. Anouchka Grose, in Chapter 3, "Gender Anxiety as a Symptom of the Analyst", re-considers Freud's treatment of the homosexual girl and criticises contemporary psychoanalysis for its dogmatism and ideological blindness, particularly in relation to contemporary gender issues. In Chapter 4, Patricia Gherovici, in "Girl, Interrupted", vividly centralises the role of the gaze in the case of a young homosexual girl and considers fresh case material as well as recent feminist and queer theory meticulously in her re-reading of the case. In Chapter 8, "Freud's Knight", Guy Le Gaufey analyses Freud's approach to the Rat Man and offers the analyst as "half the patient's symptom when the symptom has taken on its transferential value". He ponders what a psychoanalytic practice today is. Astrid Gessert in Chapter 7, "What We Can Still Learn from the Rat Man", builds a vital bridge from Freud's 1909 case to the contemporary psychoanalytic treatment of obsessional neurosis, demonstrating that modern practice must build on the foundation laid down by Freud.

There is a special relationship to language for psychotics and we must know how to work with it, notes Leon Brenner in Chapter 11, "The Form and Matter of Hallucinations in Schreber's Message Phenomena". He elaborates a Lacanian-based model for working with the phenomenon of hallucination. In Chapter 10, Rik Loose, in "The Wolf Man and Psychosis in the Post-Oedipal Era", assesses the Wolf Man case with acuity and delineates the importance of identifying and working with ordinary psychosis in today's "post-Oedipal" era. Rolf Flor's Chapter 12, in "Judge Schreber: A Neuralgic Point of Social Tensions", centralises the role of dialogical engagement with psychosis and how this differs from neuro-reductionist approaches which, he argues, were the basis of Schreber's symptoms. Annie Rogers in Chapter 9, "The Wolf Man, Invented", resplendently brings the Wolf Man to life and offers Lacan's later elaboration of the *sinthome* in her analysis of the importance of invention for the Wolf Man. Finally, Anne Worthington, in "Reading Freud's Case Studies Today", delves into what a case study is and reminds us that mass hysteria is alive and well today. As each of the contributors reminds us, the case figures – be they obsessional, hysterical, or psychotic – revive constantly in clinical work today.

There is the challenge of re-reading Freud's cases and updating them while at the same time keeping them fresh, open, and free of dogmatism, as Lacan demonstrated in his frequent re-elaborations of the cases. It is noteworthy that the contributors to this collection draw on Freud's cases not to undermine or reduce them but to advance a psychoanalysis that explores both the possibilities and the limitations of its terrain by creatively considering its theoretical and conceptual bulwarks and rendering them fit for purpose in the twenty-first century. It's helpful to keep in mind Anne Worthington's invaluable observation that the subject is not the clinical case, nor the analysand psychoanalysis itself. It is the aspiration of this collection to keep the doors of clinical practice open and not allow anachronistic dust to settle on a praxis that is up against it in our era of neuro-reductionist and cognitive behavioural ascendency.

What is psychoanalytic casework? It's a strange practice that goes something like this. It's a work of listening attentively to the ebb and flow of full and empty speech, enabling the analysand to speak within an enunciative process in which truth momentarily appears and disappears, when the important things are the most difficult to speak about, and when there is a constant interplay between rationality and irrationality. It's oriented to moments of insight and a different, perhaps even transformative structuring of the relationship to ideals and to others that can be produced by the analysand out of these gaps and irredeemable contradictions between conscious and unconscious, between analyst and analysand, between said and saying. How, we may well ask, to "re-present" this highly nuanced and valanced work outside of the clinical practice room? A case or clinical study is one mode, offering a precious window into what transpires in an analysis, demonstrating how theory is applied to practice, the unfolding of the analyst-analysand relationship, the psychoanalytic process itself. Without case studies, clinical practitioners would be lost without a compass or a guide-rope in a labyrinthine world of theory. Case studies provide essential and practical know-how and are the backbone of psychoanalytic praxis, past, present, and future. To follow Freud into that underworld of unconscious formations is to gain a special and unique access to a psychoanalytic mapping, as it is in the very movement of being drawn.

References

Forrester, John. (2016). *Thinking in Cases*. Cambridge: Polity.

Lacan, Jacques. (1953). "The Function and Field of Speech and Language in Psychoanalysis". In *Écrits: The First Complete Edition in English*, translated by Bruce Fink, pp. 197–268. New York: W.W. Norton & Co. 2006.

McGuire, William (ed.) (1974). Letter from Sigmund Freud to C. G. Jung, April 19, 1908. In *The Freud/Jung Letters: The Correspondence Between Sigmund Freud and C. G. Jung*. Princeton, NJ: Princeton University Press.

Parker, Ian. (2018). Psychoanalytic Case Presentations: The Case Against. *Lacunae, the International Journal for Lacanian Psychoanalysis*, 17, 6–36.

DORA

Fragment of an Analysis
of a Case of Hysteria

IDA BAUER

Born 1 November 1882, 32 Bergasse Strasse, Vienna
Died 21 December 1945, New York

A minuet for four characters

Freud, Sigmund. (1905). "Fragment of an Analysis
of a Case of Hysteria". In *The Standard Edition of the
Complete Psychological Works of Sigmund Freud*, translated
by James Strachey, vol. 7, pp. 1–122. London: Hogarth, 1953.

DOI: 10.4324/9781032663746-2

Chapter 1

Hysteria, History, Her Story

Freud's Dora

Olga Cox Cameron

About thirty years ago when I was beginning my psychoanalytic training, I read an interview between the great Italian novelist, Alberto Moravia, and Ireland's own great novelist, John Banville, where they foregrounded the Dora case as an almost perfect short story, more literary gem than case history. I was reminded of this moment at the start of the 2021–2022 FLi Clinical series when I heard Guy Le Gaufey being a bit tetchy about the whole idea of the case history, a view echoed in his book on this topic (Le Gaufey 2020).

It is unlikely that either Banville or Moravia had read Lacan's very first commentary on the Dora case in 1951 where he compares it to a famous seventeenth-century French novel, *La Princesse de Clèves*, revered in France as a seminal exploration of the psychology of love (Lacan [1951] 1985, 100). So Banville and Moravia were by no means the first to think like this.

It is Freud's first case history, the one he apparently agonised the most over, so much so that having submitted it for publication, he subsequently took it back and held onto it for another five years. I think it is also the only one of the case histories to be so extensively plundered for its potential as an art form, although some readers may remember that Dany Nobus showed a very good film on Freud's analysis of the Rat Man at the Psychoanalytic Film Festival in Dublin some years ago. The film, called *The Ratman* (BBC 1972), was a surprising endeavour but one that worked very well.

In contrast with that success, most of the literary re-workings of Dora I have come across have been greatly inferior to Freud's own text. Two novels, *Human Traces* by Sebastian Faulks (2005) and *The Interpretation of Murder* by Jed Rubenfield (2006) exemplify this shortfall. Both contain thinly veiled versions of Dora and her story (check out Katharina in *Human Traces*, Nora in *The Interpretation of Murder*). Both novels, however, sag somewhat under the weight of turgid and banal theorising introduced to support these accounts of hysteria. Interesting to see the case history gaining power by turning itself into a novel, while the novel loses power by turning itself into a case history.

One of Le Gaufey's reservations about the case history as a genre is its pretension to set itself up as a teaching text. In fairness, Freud absolutely does not do this with Dora. He is hyper-aware of its shortcomings, is embarrassed by them,

DOI: 10.4324/9781032663746-3

and points them out repeatedly, although four years later he is sufficiently free of this embarrassment to suggest in a footnote to the Rat Man case that a failure can actually be more fruitful than a success, since there is more to learn from it (Freud 1909, 208, fn.1).

So novel or case history? Freud most certainly does not want to write a novel, but we might note that even at the level of case history, Dora is rife with contradictory drives and internal tensions. From the outset, he made a decision not to do what most of us would like him to do; to let us see how unconscious desire pushes the story being told in particular directions – what Freud calls the interpretative work undertaken on the patient's ideas and statements. How the process occurs, how certain positions are reached is not outlined, and just giving us the results, as he so often does with Dora, makes a lot of his conclusions seem arbitrary. Freud is uneasy about this and apologises both at the beginning and at the end of the case. To let us see this as it happens would be to show "how the pure metal of valuable unconscious thoughts can be extracted from the raw material of the patient's associations" (Freud 1905, 112). This has been omitted in order to demonstrate what he calls the internal structure of hysteria, something generalised which he hopes will be of wide if not of universal import. At the end, he is unsure if he has managed to do this either, since the examination of a single case is unlikely to have fulfilled such a vast remit.

He also begins by announcing a veritable revolution in technique – a first description of free association which will become a cornerstone of psychoanalytic treatment. Having done so, Freud then appears to fall back into older habits of bossy insistence. A lot of what we see in Dora is far closer to the method described in his 1898 paper, "Sexuality in the Aetiology of the Neuroses", where he openly states that the experienced physician generally asks of his patients not elucidation but merely confirmation of his own surmises (Freud 1898, 267)! Otherwise put, the patient is told, just say, yes. Freud has no reservations at all about this level of coercion, seeing it as praiseworthy – almost intrepid – on the part of the doctor who must fearlessly require "confirmation of his surmises" (p. 266) and must overcome all resistance by *firmly insisting* on what he has inferred and by "emphasising the unshakeable nature of one's convictions" (p. 269). So there is no taking no for an answer despite the trouble this had got him into with the case of Emmy von N. (Freud 1893–1895b).

From the outset, then, there are two conflicting pulls. He would like to showcase this new method which is psychoanalysis but opts instead to demonstrate the structure of hysteria. And he has discovered free association, a revolutionary new technique, but can't quite bring himself to fully implement it.

There is also a tension – and this is evident too in *The Interpretation of Dreams* (Freud 1900a, 1900b), the sister book to the Dora case – regarding the role of the *fragment*, which he considers this case history of Dora to be: how he will come to see it with respect to the workings of the unconscious, and how he now still sees it in archaeological terms. Right now, the *fragment* is there to indicate *wholeness*. No detail fails to add up. The clue must tell the whole story, leaving no space for what Lacan will call the *mi-dit*, the half-said. So there are some boring passages in the Dora case where Freud insists on fully explaining every occurrence of a particular symptom, such as Dora's loss of voice or dragging foot. This completeness contradicts something he has already discovered although he resists this knowledge – that unconscious knowledge *is* fragmentary – a *flocculation* as Lacan calls it in *The Ethics of Psychoanalysis* ([1959–1960] 1992, 61). Freud himself in *The Interpretation of Dreams* (1900a, 1900b) speaks of fragments jammed up together like pack ice, and again much later in "Constructions in Analysis" (Freud 1937) of stand-alone fragments, fragments that do not add up. So once again, a very new insight is doing battle with an older concept, which is particularly piquant here where the *mi-dit*, the story of Dora's infatuation with Frau K., is both insistent and inarticulate.

These turbulences – not enormous but noticeable in Freud's writing of the case history – may relate to a small throw-away remark at the very beginning where he suggests that there is something inherently disturbing in neurosis itself, so maybe it is not so easy to write about it. This is a fascinating observation – Freud at his most insightful. He goes on to say that our daily habits of thought – the way we assume we know what we are talking about – make us gloss over "the bewildering character of neurosis", but this comes out again when we try to explain it (Freud 1905, 11). Maybe Freud and Le Gaufey might have found common ground!

Guy says of the case history that it is an impossible linguistic event. It is of course in all circumstances always an artefact, as Carol Owens has suggested in her Chapter 5 in this volume, "Horses for Courses: Psychoanalysis and a Small Boy". What we really want to hear is how unconscious desire deflects the story being told – how and when that happens. Ironically, generally speaking, the modalities of this process make it impossible for an outsider to listen to. We have terrific examples of very good case histories from Kristen Hennessy (Chapter 6) and Carol Owens (Chapter 5) in the present volume, but even there the actual moment-by-moment process is not simply replicated. A minimum of presentation has to occur. About two years ago, someone lent me recordings of sessions with R.D. Laing that a client had taped over several months. Sighs, silences, complaints, yawns, mutterings, unfinished sentences. It was extraordinary – as if the process itself closes itself hermetically and is available only to the participants as such. As if it can only be somewhat transmissible when fictionalised, and this tilt in the direction of fiction is non-negotiable.

Contexts: Is Dora's Hysteria Historical?

It is, I think, important to approach the concept of hysteria with a suspicious mind and to recognise that at the point Freud encountered it, it was a very specific entity to be distinguished from all of its avatars, before or since.

In our psychoanalytic vocabulary, it is the only diagnostic term not coined in the nineteenth century. The terms *psychosis* and *perversion* were invented by the relatively new science of psychiatry in the middle of that century, while it was probably Freud himself who introduced the term *obsessional neurosis*. *Hysteria* is different, it is a term with a very long history. As a disease entity, it has been described as the inscription of gender relations within medical discourse. In one nineteenth-century translation from Greek, the word *hysteria* itself is translated as *wombiness*, a condition rooted in the very nature of being female. The gender relations aspect is interesting in that what has been traditionally pathologised and is seen as primarily a feminine failing, is, broadly speaking, the propensity to be too emotional. The propensity *not to be emotional enough* was a desirable quality, something inculcated in, for example, the British educational system for boys. A touching recent advertisement on Irish television exemplifies this very sanctioned form of masculinity. A young man is on the phone to his father trying to ask the old man how he is – a question the old man is completely unable to answer. It is a very tender exchange but tells us something about the cultural milieu in which hysteria exists. Wombiness is a pathology, non-wombiness isn't.

Interestingly, hysteria as a diagnosis was actually falling into disrepute before its revival in the nineteenth century. The famous eighteenth-century English doctor, Dr. Willis, who took charge of King George III in his bouts of insanity, wrote that it was an absolute mish-mash diagnosis, a catch-all for the fantasies of ignorant doctors. When they were stumped by a symptom, they called it hysteria (Foucault 1997, 138). A statement like that would suggest that it did not have much of a future as a medical diagnosis. Weirdly, however, while, on the one hand, it was dissed by the eighteenth century as it had lost a degree of medical credibility, on the other, and at pretty much the same time, the discovery of the nervous system and the enormous impact of this discovery not just on medicine but on social life and on sentimental literature created the particular notions and definitions of hysteria that Freud was to engage with.

What the discovery of the nervous system created was a new and important intermediary zone between madness and sanity, an ambiguous zone since nervous-ness implied sensitivity, superior ability to feel, a finer type of person. As such, it gave rise to a whole range of fashionable illnesses, as well as the rest cure. This was the heyday of the protracted stay in a luxurious sanatorium, and we know that until her affair with Dora's father, Frau K. spent months of each year in one or other such place. These interludes were known as consulting Dr. Diet and Dr. Quiet – a high-class hotel in the mountain air with always the chance of a love affair with a fellow sufferer. If you remember from the case itself, Dora's father began to groan and cough and in need of better air when he needed time with Frau K, while Herr K. at the bedroom door with sex on his mind was enough to make Frau K. immediately ill, as Dora reported to Freud. Certain symptoms were privileged as episodic and incurable, and therefore very useful since they could come and go as required. Appendicitis was one such symptom and Axel Munthe (1929), a Swedish doctor who trained under Charcot, tells of the consternation among fashionable ladies in Paris when it was rumoured that American surgeons were removing appendixes. Freud has a riff in the Dora case about motives for illness but, presumably because he is living in the middle of it himself, he doesn't cite its centrality as a cultural phenomenon, although he does suggest in his 1898 paper on hysteria that the real cause of cure in these establishments is not the hydrotherapy etc. but the escape from unhappy sex lives (Freud 1898, 274). Illness then is a form of emotional currency. Specifically, nervous illness. Three of the five players in the Dora case use it to manage their sex lives.

The implication that finer nerves made for finer sensibilities and a finer type of person had another fall-out in that it ushered in a new form of writing on the body, a new way of writing sexuality, evidenced most extensively perhaps in the English novel. What Freud inherits with respect to this is perhaps a third moment. We should note that writing on the body was not a new phenomenon. Previously in Western culture it had been a religious happening. Stigmata, the wounds of Christ etched into the body, were first recorded in the thirteenth century. Holy anorexia was a feature in seventeenth-century hagiographies. These inscriptions, though primarily female, were open to either sex, but the eighteenth-century creation of the erotic body is specifically female. It was an erotic body upon which sexual desire was inscribed in the form of blushes, tears, wringing hands, and heaving bosoms, to be read by the other rather than by the subject herself. Similar to this, the hysteric writing on the body, with which Freud will engage, is an erotic inscription betraying thoughts and feelings of which the young girl is barely aware but one that speaks of sexual trauma.

The creation of this blushing tearful body was a significant re-configuration of female sexuality. In late medieval times, female desire was a dangerous force. The fifteenth-century handbook, *Malleus Maleficarum*, translated as *The Hammer of Witches*, written by two Dominican priests, speaks of insatiable female desire as the most terrible of evils (Kramer and Sprenger ([1486–1487] 2009, 121–123). By the eighteenth century, female desire is no longer audible as such, but is written on the body in this demure calligraphy, while male desire is now the privileged articulate one – uncontrollable and fierce in "unhand me, villain" scenarios!

Paradoxically, despite the blushes and the heaving bosoms, women over the course of the nineteenth century began to be viewed as essentially asexual. They were seen as intermediate between child and man – think of the child bride, Blossom, in Dickens' *David Copperfield*. I point this out because a lot of commentators joke about Freud being so defensive about discussing sex with Dora, but Henry James' (1899) novel, *The Awkward Age*, is in part about the conditions that make a girl marriageable or not and reading sexy French novels definitely put a girl out of the running. Even Françoise Dolto, a colleague of Lacan, born in 1908, recounts how her brothers were up in arms at her wanting to sit the baccalaureate because for a girl to be so educated was to be unmarriageable (Dolto 1989, 107). Freud himself has come a long way by the time he writes the Dora case. Back in 1893, when he sent "Draft B" on "The Aetiology of the Neuroses" to Fliess, he warns him to keep the manuscript away from his young wife (Masson 1985, 39).

In a very successful book, *Sex and Character*, published in 1903, Dora's era, Otto Weininger tranquilly states that "since woman possesses neither intelligence nor character her goal can only be to gratify men's desires; this is the only meaning of her life" (Ellenberger 1970, 293). There is perhaps a very faint echo of this view in the early Lacan when he says that "[a]s is true for all women the problem for Dora is fundamentally that of accepting herself as an object of desire for the man" (Lacan [1951] 1985, 99).

In this cultural milieu, it is to Freud's credit that even though he spends a lot of time barking up various wrong trees, his focus is on Dora as subject not object of desire. His question is, "who is she in love with?" This remains true even when it shades into being a non-question since he himself has already answered it.

Wombiness may still be a problem today but assuredly it is not the problem it was back then. Everything about female sexuality was problematised to the point that books were written on how to keep young girls on vegetarian diets with frequent icy baths in order to delay puberty. Excessive female desire could cause sterility and was to be discouraged and curtailed (Stone 1977, 676). In any era, the question of what it is to be a sexed being is enormous but how do you either ask or answer it if you are by definition asexual – an identity not chosen but mandated by the Other.

I am leaning on the historical context to show that hysteria at that point occupied a very specific place. To an unparalleled degree it is true to its name *hysteria* – the problems you face when you have a womb. Unsurprisingly in this era, if women are the problem, then men will be the ones who seek and perhaps provide solutions. Charcot demonstrated the stages of hysteria on the woman's body, Freud listened to and recorded the woman hysteric – a kind of *women show and men tell* scenario. What I like about some of these accounts are the power ploys of the powerless. According to Munthe (1929), Charcot's trainee, many of the hysterics in the Salpêtrière rehearsed their performances before providing theatrical demonstrations of Charcot's (erroneous) three stages of hysteria for the impressed medics at his Friday lectures. Anna O. (Freud 1893–1895a) ran rings round Breuer, had him there for hours at a time twice a day, could only recognise him when he held her hands and eventually brought this intense phantom love affair to a climax by giving birth to his phantom child. Emmy von N. (Freud 1893–1895b), bullied by Freud into having all her painful memories erased by hypnosis, outfoxes him, not so much by rebellion as by over-compliance, seemingly forgetting everything – her marriage, her children, her whole life – leaving Freud worried that he has perhaps overshot the mark! Even Dora's disregarded and despised mother manages to wield her scrubbing brush in such a way as to make life impossible for her family. As Foucault pointed out in his introduction to *The History of Sexuality*, power is very often a two-way street (1976, 12).

Lastly with respect to this very specific era, there is the question of masturbation. An anonymous publication in 1716 called *Onania* (*Masturbation*) had an absolutely enormous influence – completely ludicrously – on both medicine and general culture (Anonymous [1716] 2010). It was seen as the worst of all possible vices, ruining health both physical and mental, causing blindness, pallor, and as one tract put it, this was obvious to everyone because of the lean and shaky shanks of those who practised it. If a girl had vaginal thrush, it was an indication of masturbation

– you can see this in the Dora case. This constitutes an alarming example of how a ridiculous theory can run the show and run it very harmfully. It was seen as a cause of madness and appears in late nineteenth-century clinical textbooks as a distinct nosological entity; masturbational insanity (Bynum, Shepherd, and Porter 1988, 87). At the time of writing the Dora case, Freud was still an adherent of this theory but changed his mind soon afterwards. We can smile at this madness, but we would be very innocent and very naive not to wonder if at least some of the theories we hold dear will not be laughing stocks in a few years' time. The problem of course is to know which ones!

But Maybe Not Just Historical?

All of this – the role of illness, the dangers of masturbation, the problematisation of every phase of female sexuality, creates a world that is markedly different to our own, and yet the Dora case can also very validly be read as ultra-modern – a narrative of something only recently highlighted and for which there wasn't even a name back then – *gaslighting*! The kick-off for Dora's analysis is not the event by the lake with Herr K. but the fact that the three others conspire to see this as a figment of her imagination. It would be to do less than justice to the Dora case as a great short story if one were to blinker oneself to its many interwoven threads, but it is important to see the gaslighting narrative as the simplest, most direct, most un-deviating diegetic thrust, the one that opens and closes what we read. Freud, even though he is pursuing a narrative of his own, makes that clear.

Freud believes Dora – the only one who does so apart perhaps from her mother. He spells out very clearly the fact of gaslighting as the reason Dora is with him. He remarks repeatedly on the fact that what enrages and embitters her most is this, and what marks her cure at the end is breaking through the lie and getting all three to acknowledge the truth of what happened. He spells out for us the exact time frame of the two events, noting that initially when Dora told her mother about Herr K.'s sexual approach at the lake, the story stands, and is not as such refuted.

Herr K. is perturbed, respectful, offering to come in person to explain. It is only some weeks later that his attitude completely changes. Armed with the information that she has been reading about sex – something no respectable girl should be doing – he suggests, to the father's evident relief, that she has made the whole thing up. The father very clearly tells Freud that this was when Dora's symptoms took off.

It is quite possible that a twenty-first-century analyst, alert to such wrongs, would hear only the gaslighting and nothing else. One of the reasons it is tempting to read Dora as a short story is the way Freud lays out this narrative so clearly and then leapfrogs over it to tell his own story. Another is the manner in which this blindness serves him so well. If this were a Netflix drama, a major turning point would occur here. But Freud drives straight on through. In pursuit of his own narrative, he never asks, "what does it do to someone to be gaslighted?" Only at the very end – because, for all his misconceptions, he is honest – can we wonder: *what is it to be gaslighted by the one you love?*

What Freud produces here is a brilliant Sherlock Holmes pounce: "Why now?" "How come this situation worked just fine for so long?"

Before we follow Freud onto the new terrain opened up by this question, we might note that the gaslighting episode chimes exactly with one of Lacan's definitions of hysteria. As you can see in the Dora case, for Freud, the writing on the body is the definitive mark of hysteria – it is what distinguishes it from other neuroses. But other definitions exist. One in particular has always pleased me. In his fifth seminar, *The Formations of the Unconscious*, Lacan describes the hysteric as finding it difficult to establish a relation with the Other, constituted as bearer of the spoken sign, in which she can hold onto her own place as subject (Lacan 1957–1958, 343). I find this to be a blisteringly true statement. If you have been corralled into a given place by the Other, how do you escape since everything you do and say will confirm an already fixed view? The protest of the so-called hysteric is simply further proof of her hysteria. In the world in which Dora grows up, *Woman* is very explicitly a male construct, positioned in the symbolic order in such a way as to make it difficult for her to hold on to her place as subject. As late as the 1950s, the "trauma" of eventlessness could still be invoked as a defining feature of female existence. So Lacan's definition covers a very wide spectrum, but it is also ultra-relevant to the gaslighting drama that kicks off Dora's treatment and to the manner in which she eventually cures herself.

So back to Freud's harsh yet brilliant question, "Why now?"

Symptom or *Sinthome*?

In a very interesting article back in 1994, Paul Verhaeghe suggests that people come to analysis because their symptom has stopped working, and I wonder if this is what happened here (1994, 48). As Verhaeghe says, the symptom ensures a kind of stability for the subject, and it is only when this stabilising function has been impaired that the subject seeks help. With marked frequency in these years, Freud insisted that the symptom as such *is* the subject's sex life. To quote just one example; in a paper written in 1905, the same year as the publication of the Dora case, he states, "hysteria is the expression of a peculiar behaviour of the individual's sexual function" (Freud 1906 [1905], 273), adding; "*the patient's symptoms represent his sexual activity*" (p. 278, original emphasis).

In line with this view, he reads Dora's throat problems as her identification with and semi-enactment of the oral sex that is her father's sex life with Frau K. But perhaps we might broaden our definition of the symptom here to consider Lacan's later definition which is the symptom as *sinthome*. This is a kind of cobbled together solution to the difficulties inherent in the fundamental fantasy,[1] but which, against the odds perhaps, permits the subject to live a version of unconscious desire. The strange but apparently quite stable scenario that Freud uncovers at the end of Dora's first telling of her story could very well be her *sinthome* in this Lacanian sense.

To me, this makes for a much more interesting version of the symptom as the subject's mode of living sexual desire than Freud's rather conflicted attempts to make each bodily manifestation carry part of an originating trauma. He is very keen on this theory in these years and really wants the symptom to provide specific evidence of something hidden, in the same way as a shard of pottery could tell something important and exact about an earlier era. He had taken this hope to slightly ridiculous extremes in *Studies in Hysteria* (Freud 1893–1895a, 1893–1895b, 1893–1895c) when he ascribed one set of conflictual memories to the pains in one leg of Elisabeth von R. while a whole other set were represented by the pains in the other leg. Here he spends several pages quarrelling with himself trying to find an exact psychical origin for pains and aches which he suspects may actually be bodily in origin – which in Dora is "somatic compliance" (Freud 1905, 40).

Seeing the sexual quartet that works for Dora as her *sinthome* in the Lacanian sense makes for a reading that is not just more interesting but more novelistic. As Eve and Helena indicate in the FLi Series Preface, we do not want to be dogmatic about the case histories but to ask questions about them and perhaps also to play a little with them.

Odd though this originating scenario may look, it works for Dora. She is an active participant in a strange sexual foursome. Frau K. and her father carry on undisturbed with Dora acting as babysitter to give them plenty of time together. She herself and Herr K. hang out in what looks like a kind of desexualised sexual relationship – something like courtly love, where she is showered with flowers, gifts, attention, spending a lot of time alone with him. However, these two heterosexual imbroglios are surface events – the erotic core is Dora's infatuation with Frau K.

Henry James could do great things with this kind of situation. Freud himself was uncomfortably aware of its novelistic tilt, even saying that if it really was a novel, he would have left the best bits out such as Dora and Frau K. talking sex at night in their shared bedroom in order to keep Herr K. and his sexual urges on the other side of the locked door! (Freud 1905, 61). If this criss-cross of erotic tension is Dora's sex life, how did it come about? Clearly certain transmutations had to occur. Initially Dora was part of the general indignation regarding the scandalously obvious affair between her father and Frau K. She even took it upon herself to reproach him, being absolutely unconvinced by the ridiculous story with which the father tried to cover it up (p. 38). And initially, as we saw at 14 years old, she was genuinely alarmed by the snatched kiss from him (pp. 27–28), evidence of male desire, and for a time made sure never to be alone with him. But then what happened and why? Freud's desire to be scientifically thorough, to explain everything to the reader is oddly countermanded by the very novelistic omissions that sustain the erotic tension in this story.

The scenario that established itself lets us see how extraordinarily varied are the ways in which one can have a sex life. And so we should be asking: which of the components of this scenario are operative for Dora's sex life? Freud tells us repeatedly that the most consistently repressed element in the entire story – presumably its erotic core for Dora – is the sex talk at night with Frau K. But does Herr K., forlornly hovering outside the door, heighten the thrill? Interestingly, Dora, who is hyper-sensitive to any notion of being used, does not at all mind her role here, telling Freud that this is Frau K.'s way of avoiding sex with her husband. Although Freud jumps to the wrong conclusion, he may not have been wrong in seeing that Herr K. played a pivotal sexual role. The penis/phallus lurking in the wings seems to be an essential player. When it emerges from the wings, however, it creates real panic. We see this in the earlier episode of attempted seduction by Herr K. of Dora when she was 14 (pp. 27–28). We have no idea if Freud is correct in surmising that Dora felt Herr K.'s erect penis pressing against her when he grabbed and kissed her (p. 29), and we question his confident assumption that a normal girl would have been excited by this. But we can see that Dora was very much alarmed, cancelling an outing with the K.'s after that, and avoiding being alone with this man. She also became phobic about male arousal and would not pass a man in excited conversation with a woman on the street. While Freud is crass in thinking that her not being excited by the kiss is abnormal, indeed hysterical, I do think the ensuing phobia is noteworthy. Herr K. at the bedroom door is Herr K. looking for sex. Herr K. going to bed with the governess is Herr K. looking for and getting sex. Dora is not bothered by any of this and has no hesitation in being alone with him. However, when she herself is directly approached sexually by Herr K., everything falls apart.

So we have a rather extraordinary sexual scenario – an impotent penis and a potent one – both somehow sustaining the *jouissance* of two women in bed talking sex.[2] We don't know what the other three made of this situation, but it seems that it worked just fine as Dora's *sinthome*.

Is part of what holds the symptom together for Dora her own position as Madonna in this relationship? Remember the second dream and its associations (pp. 94–111), the two hours she spends in dreamy contemplation of the Madonna (p. 96), and the way Lacan links this to her question "what is it to be a woman?", which he to some extent also sees as the basis of her adoration of Frau K. (Lacan [1951] 1985, 97–98). Everything we read about her relationship with Herr K. – the daily flowers, the gifts, the letters, the hours spent in his company – could remind us of the Lady and the chaste lover in courtly love. Herr K. upends all of this with a direct sexual approach, adding insult to injury by making it the exact same approach he had used with the governess – Dora is just another girl. I have to say I find the approach of Herr K. astonishingly unseductive. Not "I can't stop thinking about you. You are so beautiful" but "I get nothing out of her. What about you?" Like a supermarket. No rice there. What about the other one? Really? How many people would find this overwhelmingly persuasive?

Both Freud and Lacan ask who Herr K. is for Dora. While Lacan's answer is brilliant, and brilliantly analytical, I am not sure if it entirely covers the ground. He vaults us back to a foundational moment in Dora's babyhood where she sits on the floor sucking her thumb while pulling rhythmically on her brother's earlobe (p. 98). Lacan sees this as the imaginary matrix that will shape all the later situations in her life – a statement that sounds like a precursor of what he will develop later as the fundamental fantasy. He is trenchant here: "it gives the measure of what woman and man signify for her now. Woman is the object of desire, linked to a primitive oral desire, and yet in which she must come to recognise her own genital nature"

(p. 98). It seems that, for both Freud and Lacan, desiring a woman can only be masculine. Neither of them takes on board that a woman can desire a woman. So, for Lacan, this foundational scene "shows us that her only opening to the object was through the intermediary of the masculine partner" (p. 98).

Hard not to be impressed by what Lacan infers from this early scene. He may well be correct, but equally these two instances of masculinist bias – a woman can be desired only from a masculine position, and a woman must come to terms with her position as an object of desire – may have inflected his insights in questionable directions.

What is Dora's relation to male sexuality? While her response to the kiss is not hysterical, the ensuing phobia appears very extreme. Some intense fright/refusal is at work here. And then there is the missing step in Freud's account. We know that initially regarding her father's affair, Dora was part of the indignation brigade and took him to task. What had to happen to make her the mainstay in what has now expanded into a foursome sustained by very specific criss-crossings of sexual enjoyment?

If the scenario that worked is Dora's *sinthome*, the event that destabilised it is the scene by the lake (Freud 1905, 25–26) which at some level replicates the kiss at age 14. This is not a guess. Dora herself makes the connection. But why was it so much more catastrophic and what might have remedied it? Again, this is Dora's own question. Even after telling, this situation was not without remedy. Herr K. would come in person to sort out any misunderstanding. At that point, something Dora was hoping for did not happen. Check out her admission when Freud is questioning her about this:

> You…thought your accusation might be a means of inducing him to travel to the place where you were living.— 'As he actually offered to do at first,' Dora threw in[3]—'In that way your longing for him might have been appeased'—here she nodded assent, a thing I had not expected—'and he might have made you the amends you desired.'
>
> (Freud 1905, 107)

And the blade that severs these conjoined narratives is the unknown answer to the question Dora then asks, "What amends?" (Freud 1905, 107).

If we consider the narratives that make up the *sinthome* as forming an inner and an outer circle, the inner circle is Dora and Frau K. in the bedroom talking sex, and the outer one is the banished potent penis and presumably the impotent one. The kiss and the lake scene target the outer circle. Both are clearly extremely disturbing, but what smashes the entire *sinthome* is the destruction of the inner one brought about by Frau K.'s betrayal. And Freud gets that.

A very interesting question opened up by the Dora case is that of the usefulness of a failed analysis. The two dreams mark the point where Dora opts to opt out, and so solicit our special attentiveness in their own right, but also with respect to Dora's assessment of the analysis as not worth going on with. We can of course only play with these dreams since we are not in either the transferential or counter-transferential situation in which they occur. But playing can be useful.

Dora's Dreams

We know that her first dream (Freud 1905, 64) coincided with Dora's decision to leave the analysis. We also know that she left in much better shape than at the start. If we stay with Lacan's definition in Seminar V cited earlier, she actually overcomes the dilemma of the hysteric since she becomes able to hold on to her place as subject and to take the correct actions. This in itself is remarkable, since she could easily have been crushed or helplessly outraged by this second manifestation of adult blindness – this insistent masculinist discourse blotting out her own story.

I read both dreams as referencing female desire. In the first dream, both the manifest content and two of the first three associations refer to conflict between the parents in which the mother's desire is overwritten, and in the egregious bracelet anecdote her rightful fury is explicit (p. 69).

What the woman wants is irrelevant. Giving the gift of jewellery might look like an act of love and recognition, but only the man's wishes count. Similarly, for Dora herself, there is no way the father will not ride roughshod over her wishes in pursuit of his own desires, no way Frau K. will not give her over in favour of the man. Do these cruel facts perforate her fantasy of her role as that of the indispensable one, the one who facilitated and sustained the whole situation? This is something I have seen a few times in my work – how utterly devastating it can be to discover that one is not the linchpin, if that is where you have pitched your life. Remember Anna Livia's last speech in *Finnegans Wake* as she-Liffey-flows into the sea: "Thinking always if I go all goes" (Joyce [1939] 1992, 627). And also, is Dora's persistence in pursuing this impossible demand an effective means of enacting the dilemma of the hysteric?

Initially Freud does very well on the first dream. He follows the directions set forth in *The Interpretation of Dreams*, taking each segment piece by piece, since the overall narrative is what we do with the fragments that go into creating the dream, while also as Freud notes, being sometimes a carrier of the intensities propelling it.

Freud picks up on a really interesting condensation – the father at her bedside rescuing her which is exactly what he will not do. And, of course, neither will Freud. A double image carrying too the threat of Herr K.'s sexuality. Did Freud really and very brilliantly recognise why this dream of rescue/threat occurred at exactly this point in Dora's analysis? In a footnote, he quotes himself telling Dora that the reason the dream has recurred now is because she needs to rescue herself from the analysis and has decided to leave (Freud 1905, 70, fn. 2). I wonder if this really happened, since presumably it would have had a huge bearing on all that followed. Indeed, Freud himself seems to admit as much at the end. Telling us that he actually said it then marks an odd moment in this case where Freud is so frank about his mistakes. And the place at which he locates this interpretation is novelistically brilliant – a footnote inserted at the point of his most dogmatic insistence that Dora is in love with Herr K. – creating a chiasmus where his most passionate misreading collides with his most perceptive insight.

While Freud accomplishes a number of extraordinarily perceptive moves in his analysis of this first dream, very many of the concatenations he elaborates are his own readings and not Dora's. Note the number of times he says he had to supply the rest himself, admitting at one point that he has been "framing conjectures and filling in deficiencies" (p. 85). There is a sense that his thrust to do this, to fill in deficiencies, is theory-driven. He is keen to back up his recent theoretical discoveries, in particular those of *The Interpretation of Dreams*. Hence the riff on wish fulfilment, but as we now know, "Beyond the Pleasure Principle" (Freud 1920) greatly modifies this position.

But although Freud sounds somewhat coercive from the start, there is a definite sense that he and Dora are working together on the dream until, rather unexpectedly, he takes off on his own. Bringing in a table with a box of matches on it, a weird move that Dora actually doesn't even notice (Freud 1905, 71), sets him off on a series of interpretations, moving from bedwetting to masturbation and from there to thrush, syphilis, and a pasting on of the Oedipus complex to explain dyspnoea (pp. 71–93).

As he himself admits, this suite of ideas is predominantly his, not Dora's, reminding me of a recent analysand, who would throw himself on the couch, recount his dream, and loftily instruct me, "Freud away on that now!"

Despite this rather egregious overwriting of Dora's own story, I find Freud impressive in working with both of Dora's dreams. In the second dream (p. 94), he stays closer to the text and his reading gains from being less theory-driven. He is again clearly guided by his own recommendations in *The Interpretation of Dreams*, starting with the day's events which may have stimulated the dream (Freud 1900b, 555). He is of course not in a position to read these events – Dora's questions – "why did I keep silent?", then "why did I tell?" – as pertaining to her decision to do exactly the same to him. This dream is particularly interesting in that the initial text opens out into crucial intercalations brought about by Freud's attempts at interpretation. Freud notes in "Now he is dead, and if you like you can come" an addendum of there having been a question mark after the word "like" (Freud 1905, 94, fn. 2), reminding Dora of a letter from Frau K. As mentioned earlier, I read in both dreams something about female desire. Here the question mark in the middle of the sentence "Now he is dead, and if you like? you can come" is a woman offering choice – "if you like?" This contrasts sharply with the impositional insistence to which Dora is now being subjected. Significantly and fatally Freud leaps straight over this interjection to get back to what he sees as the real business – the scene at the lake.

Dora's abrupt departure curtails interpretation, but Freud astutely notes the prevalence of the signifier "picture" in the dream (p. 99, fn.1). Quite an extensive exploration of the gaze could be undertaken here, focussing not just on the two hours contemplating the Madonna but also the calm reading of the big book – initially repressed but then retrieved in the associative chain – and as such marked by Freud as the most valuable part of dreams (1933, 25). In both of these instances, the gaze is Dora's. She is subject, not object.

Curiously, all through this dream runs the theme of aloneness, initially pervaded with anxiety, as she carries out her decision to go on alone. But she is ultimately serene and self-possessed as she settles to look at what she wants to see in the big book.

Conclusion

How would a novelist end this story? The gaslighting narrative which Dora finds for herself without any help from her elders offers satisfactory closure, but what novelist could have invented the coda provided by real life? We are told that Dora later became a champion bridge player, with for a partner, guess who? Frau K.!

As psychoanalysts we are well aware that every reading is a misreading. Freud's is obvious even to himself. But if, as Lacan says, all truth has the structure of fiction, I would hope that playing with the case histories as we have been doing here can be a way of unearthing the alternative readings that lurk inside all our stories.

Notes

1 Lacan's algorithm for this concept is actually helpful, ($ ◊ o). The subject, barred by her encounter with crucial limitation, is caught up in relation of pursuit/avoidance – lozenge – to that which drives her desire – o. For all of us, the life we live is inflected/deflected by this unconscious underlay.
2 Lacan's use of the term *jouissance* is both difficult to describe and relatively accessible. It denotes the addictive enjoyment – not necessarily pleasurable – that drives us to repeat familiar forms of suffering and to require specific conditions in our love life.
3 Note the joint narrative here.

References

Anonymous. (1716). *Onania: Or, the Heinous Sin of Self-pollution, and All its Frightful Consequences, in Both Sexes*. Gale ECCO, 2010. BBC (British Broadcasting Corporation). (1972). *The Ratman*. Television program. Written and produced by Bruce Norman.
Bynum, William. F., Shepherd, Michael, and Porter, Roy (eds). (1988). *The Anatomy of Madness*, vol. 3. London. Routledge.
Dolto, Françoise. (1989). *Autoportrait d'une Psychanalyste*. Paris: Seuil.
Ellenberger, Henry. (1970). *The Discovery of the Unconscious: The History and Evolution of Dynamic Psychiatry*. New York: Basic Books.
Faulks, Sebastian. (2005). *Human Traces*. London: Hutchinson.
Foucault, Michel. (1976). *The History of Sexuality*, vol. 1. London: Penguin.
Foucault, Michel. (1997). *Madness and Civilization*. London: Routledge.
Freud, Sigmund. (1893–1895a). "Fräulein Anna. O". In *The Standard Edition of the Complete Psychological Works of Sigmund Freud*, translated by James Strachey, vol. 2, pp. 21–47. London: Hogarth, 1955.
Freud, Sigmund. (1893–1895b). "Frau Emmy von N". In *The Standard Edition of the Complete Psychological Works of Sigmund Freud*, translated by James Strachey, vol. 2, pp. 48–105. London: Hogarth, 1955.

Freud, Sigmund. (1893–1895c). "Katharina". In *The Standard Edition of the Complete Psychological Works of Sigmund Freud*, translated by James Strachey, vol. 2, pp. 125–134. London: Hogarth, 1955.

Freud, Sigmund. (1898). "Sexuality in the Aetiology of the Neuroses". In *The Standard Edition of the Complete Psychological Works of Sigmund Freud*, translated by James Strachey, vol. 3, pp. 263–286. London: Hogarth, 1955.

Freud, Sigmund. (1900a). "The Interpretation of Dreams". In *The Standard Edition of the Complete Psychological Works of Sigmund Freud*, translated by James Strachey, vol. 4. London: Hogarth, 1955.

Freud, Sigmund. (1900b). "The Interpretation of Dreams". In *The Standard Edition of the Complete Psychological Works of Sigmund Freud*, translated by James Strachey, vol. 5. London: Hogarth 1955.

Freud, Sigmund. (1905). "Fragment of an Analysis of a Case of Hysteria". In *The Standard Edition of the Complete Psychological Works of Sigmund Freud*, translated by James Strachey, vol. 7, pp. 7–122. London: Hogarth, 1955.

Freud, Sigmund. (1906 [1905]). "My Views on the Part Played by Sexuality in the Aetiology of the Neuroses". In *The Standard Edition of the Complete Psychological Works of Sigmund Freud*, translated by James Strachey, vol. 7, pp. 271–279. London: Hogarth, 1955.

Freud, Sigmund. (1909). "Notes Upon a Case of Obsessional Neurosis". In *The Standard Edition of the Complete Psychological Works of Sigmund Freud*, translated by James Strachey, vol. 10, pp. 151–249. London: Hogarth, 1955.

Freud, Sigmund. (1920) "Beyond the Pleasure Principle". In *The Standard Edition of the Complete Psychological Works of Sigmund Freud*, translated by James Strachey, vol. 18, pp. 7–64. London: Hogarth, 1955.

Freud, Sigmund. (1933). "Revision of the Theory of Dreams: New Introductory Lectures on Psychoanalysis". In *The Standard Edition of the Complete Psychological Works of Sigmund Freud*, translated by James Strachey, vol. 22, pp. 7–30. London: Hogarth, 1955.

Freud, Sigmund. (1937). "Constructions in Analysis". In *The Standard Edition of the Complete Psychological Works of Sigmund Freud*, translated by James Strachey, vol. 23, pp. 257–269. London: Hogarth, 1955.

James, Henry. (1899). *The Awkward Age*. London: Heinemann.

Joyce, James. (1939). *Finnegans Wake*. London: Penguin, 1992.

Kramer, Heinrich and Sprenger, Jacob. (1486–1487). *The Hammer of Witches*. Cambridge: Cambridge University Press, 2009.

Lacan, Jacques. (1951). "Intervention on Transference". In *In Dora's Case*, edited by Charles Bernheimer and Claire Kahane, pp. 92–104. New York: Columbia Press, 1985.

Lacan, Jacques. (1957–1958). *Formations of the Unconscious*. In *The Seminar of Jacques Lacan, Book V*, translated by Russell Grigg. Cambridge: Polity Press, 1997.

Lacan, Jacques. (1959–1960). *The Ethics of Psychoanalysis*. In *The Seminar of Jacques Lacan, Book VII*, translated by Denis Porter, edited by Jacques-Alain Miller. New York: Norton, 1992.

Le Gaufey, Guy. (2020). *Le cas en psychanalyse*. Paris. Kindle.

Masson, Jeffrey. M. (ed.) (1985). *The Complete Letters of Sigmund Freud to Wilhelm Fliess (1987–1904)*. London: Belknap Press.

Munthe, Axel. (1929). *The Story of Saint Michele*. London: Murray.

Rubenfeld, Jed. (2006). *The Interpretation of Murder*. London: Picador.

Stone, Lawrence. (1977). *The Family: Sex and Marriage in England, 1500–1800*. London: HarperCollins.

Verhaeghe, Paul. (1994). "Psychotherapy, Psychoanalysis and Hysteria". *The Letter: Lacanian Perspectives on Psychoanalysis*, 2, 47–68.

Chapter 2

Return to Dora, Again and Again

Jamieson Webster

Why do we return to the case of Dora again and again? Indeed, why did Lacan? How can it be that after decades of work on Dora there is still more to learn from this case of a teenage girl at the turn of the century? Lacan turns to Freud's "Fragment of an Analysis of a Case of Hysteria" (1905) every time he re-elaborates aspects of his thinking. In fact, Lacan called himself an hysteric, walking about on stage speaking, performing, clowning around, not knowing what he was saying or where he was going. He placed his audience into the role of the analyst-listener:

> Freud's text on Dora … is even more astounding for the double face it presents. On the one hand there are the weaknesses and inadequacies that strike novices as the first items to be pointed up, but on the other hand there is the depth that is reached by everything Freud comes up against, revealing to what extent he was right there, turning around the very field we are trying to map out.
>
> (Lacan [1972–1973] 1999, 108)

Lacan sought to demonstrate what was possible through a progressive *hystericisation* of speech, meaning a forceful interrogation of desire – this depth that Dora brings. I think Dora will always be important for psychoanalysis, to reignite desire for listening to the conundrums of desire, to re-find our co-ordinates that we map and remap with every patient.

"Intervention on Transference" was published in 1966 in the *Écrits* (Lacan [1951] 2006, 176–185) where it is noted that the text is based on an earlier one Lacan presented at a psychoanalytic congress in 1951. He reads Freud's Dora case as unfolding dialectically, step by step. The momentum of the case breaks down where Freud's countertransference appears, leaving him blind. Lacan nevertheless feels that the case concludes with a degree of dignity restored to Dora, who gets those around her to acknowledge what she understood through her work with Freud.

Freud, Lacan says, will not tolerate the complaint of the beautiful soul who bemoans a disorder they fail to see in themselves. This is the first dialectical reversal, Freud asking Dora: *what is your part in the disorder you complain of?* Through her dreams they discover that she had protected the affair between her father and

DOI: 10.4324/9781032663746-4

Frau K. that she was now trying to sabotage. In fact, she seems to have made herself its linchpin, and why she abandoned this role is unclear to her. This revelation brings Freud to a second dialectical turn. *Whom does Dora serve? Whom does she protect?*

Frau K. had in fact betrayed Dora the most bitterly and brutally, giving to her husband the trump card to use against Dora to deny her claims regarding her husband's sexual advances. And yet, Dora maintained an attachment to Frau K., refusing to reveal to Freud some of the secrets of their relationship. What was the nature of Dora's interest in Frau K.? This could have led, Lacan claims, to a third dialectical turning point, opening the door not to an object, but a mystery: the mystery of Dora's femininity. This is what is figured in the image of Dora stunned for two hours in front of the Sistine Madonna whose virginal face is also the image of horror before the crucifixion of her own child. An image of plenitude and loss.

Lacan contrasts this image with another image from her childhood – what he calls the limit of Dora's question in a matrix, an imago, of what man and woman mean to her. Lacan sees in this childhood image of *Dora sucking her thumb and tugging on her brother's ear*, "an imaginary mold in which all the situations orchestrated by Dora during her lifetime came to be cast" (Lacan [1951] 2006, 180). She will proceed principally along the two vectors encapsulated in this image; by means of the orality signalled in the *sucking*, and by means of the *tugging* on the masculine, signalled in the borrowing of her brother's ear. This *imaginary mold* will serve her in recasting what is problematic: *Why* the father-daughter/mother-son split in the family? *How* to locate herself in these couplets? *How* to regain the love of her Father from his mistress? Even Dora's image of her body, fragmenting under conflict, will be sustained by the sucking and the tugging, via oral symptoms, from the coughing to the loss of her voice, to the image of oral sex, and via a dependence on the actual presence of a masculine partner, which is partly why Herr K. was for so long tolerated.

Important for Lacan is the fact that she is coming closer to what he calls *ideal images*, the stereotypes of love which Freud woefully participated in. Such proximity brings with it a suddenly anxious wavering in the hysterical subject, which is a means of possible dispersal of these images. Dora suddenly shuts the door on Freud at this point, leaving him on the threshold of her mystery. But having done so, she taught Freud a lesson on transference. This is also the threshold Dora is pushing up against – the limits to what is possible in a culture that repudiates female sexuality. Lacan names this threshold the real. Freud's ability to let her take him there is the reason why the Dora case continues to remain so utterly contemporary – she is always to be found at the limit.

Turning to technique, in Lacan's first seminar from 1953–1954, *Book I: Freud's Papers on Technique*, he states what the process of analysis consists of: we break the moorings of speech, allowing the subject to see the diverse parts of the self-image procuring a maximal narcissistic projection. Freud, he says, intervenes at the place where chaos and aborted identifications composed Dora's life. Freud isn't able, according to Lacan, to integrate her desire on the symbolic plane. Instead, he was fascinated with imaginary aspects of the case, repeatedly telling her she loves her father and Herr K. If Freud had been able to say, "you love Frau K.," she would have been able to at least move more willingly in her direction. Not as an endpoint, not as a realisation of love, but as the next dialectical turn.

In Lacan's third seminar in 1955–1956, *The Psychoses*, he surprisingly returns to Dora after going into great depth on Schreber. He tries to understand the difference between persecutory thoughts in psychosis versus hysteria. Lacan begins:

> The history, as you know, is that of a minuet for four characters, Dora, her father, Herr K. and Frau K. Dora in fact uses Herr K as her ego, in that it is by means of him that she is effectively able to support her relationship with Frau K … It's only Herr K's mediation that enables Dora to sustain a bearable relationship. While this mediating fourth person is essential for maintaining the situation, this is not because the object of her affection is the same sex as herself, but because she has the most profoundly motivated relations of identification and rivalry with her father, further accentuated by the fact that the mother is a person completely obliterated in the parental couple.
>
> (Lacan [1955–1956] 1993, 91)

Lacan finds in the Dora case the instigating event, the fertile moment, which he ties more to speech acts than a reference, or emphasis, on given events in reality, namely, when Herr K. says to Dora, "My wife means nothing to me."[1] "Everything," Lacan says, "then happened as if she had answered to him – *So, what can you be to me, then?*" (p. 91, emphasis Lacan). Here you see her leaning on her identification with the male partner, ego to ego, and her reply is the inverted form of the other's saying. This is contrasted with Schreber's instigating thought – *it must be very nice to be a woman undergoing intercourse* – in identification with the opposite sex.

After this moment at the lake, Dora suddenly began making demands, declaring that her father wanted to "prostitute her and surrender her to Herr K. in exchange for maintaining his ambiguous relation with the latter's wife" (p. 92). Freud even remarks that she herself understood that this was somewhat of an exaggeration, but she could sometimes think of nothing else. Freud calls this a super-valent thought designed to block out all others and obscure some truth. This is important for understanding the kind of demands or even allegations that can arise in a treatment; the persecutory feelings aroused by collapsing ego-identifications in hysterogenic events, according to Lacan.

Lacan notes that some kind of distance, or mediation, that had helped Dora, collapsed. Her paranoiac thoughts were designed to re-establish a necessary space. Sometimes this took on an actual form such as compulsively running away from these three figures, her father, Herr K., and Frau K. At other times, a distance is established by dreaming of revenge against her father and separating him from his mistress, or, eventually, after taking some actual distance from the affairs, desiring to establish the obfuscated truth of what was taking place among the four parties.

The Freudian topography of the ego shows us how an hysteric (or an obsessional) "uses his or her ego in order to raise the question, that is, precisely in order not to raise it" (p. 174). Yet, the signifier insists. Dora, he says, is wondering – what is a woman? In the work with Freud, she is attempting to construct a position for herself. But she keeps getting lost in her identifications with men:

> Her identification with the man, bearer of the penis, is for her on this occasion a means of approaching this definition that escapes her. She literally uses the penis as an imaginary instrument for apprehending what she hasn't succeeded in symbolizing ... Becoming a woman and wondering what a woman is are two essentially different things. I would go even further – it's because one doesn't become one that one wonders and, up to a point, to wonder is the contrary of becoming one.
>
> (Lacan [1955–1956] 1993, 178)

Ultimately, the symbolic does not offer answers for the most pressing questions around life as such: death, sex, especially sexed reproduction, and madness. One might suspect this is why Freud said that to wonder about the meaning of life is to already be neurotic. Lacan emphasises the point of lack in the symbolic, the failure with respect to any answer, which the hysteric, he notes, targets with precision.

The difference between psychosis and hysteria at this place of encounter is important: the aim of psychosis is to insist on meaning because the encounter with lack in the Other truly obliterates them, while the neurotic insists on their question, ultimately an inhibition with encountering lack. With psychosis, the worry is always the potential violence that can erupt from needing to insist on their delusion. With neurosis, we struggle to clear a path from wondering – and all its attendant symptoms – to becoming, desiring.

Becoming Dora

Lacan deepens this notion of becoming in Seminar IV from 1956–1957, *The Object Relation.* He notes that Dora and the young female homosexual in Freud's "The Psychogenesis of a Case of Homosexuality in a Woman" (1920) bear the same structure of subject-father-lady. The lady represents for the young female homosexual an important beyond, an Other, a point of address and questioning. Yet, the cases differ insofar as Dora is after *the father's love*, while the young female homosexual seeks *the gift of the Father* or his object. The lady, Frau K., is a placeholder for Dora as the subject, while the lady is the object (cause) of desire for the young female homosexual.

The young female homosexual seems to want to teach the father, showing him in an exhibitionistic fashion her selfless love for the lady. When she is rejected by both, she rushes to commit suicide. Dora, on the other hand, sustains her symptom and her questions, even, remarkably, after Frau K. ruthlessly rejects her. As Lacan says of Dora and the hysteric more generally:

> The subject is interested in the situation as such, that is to say, in the relations of desire ... which remains a question mark, an x, an enigma, which the symptom cloaks itself in ... the mark of a special signifier, a chosen signifier, which here happens to be an obligatory path which, as it were, the course of the vital force, desire in this case, must follow.
>
> (Lacan [1957–1958] 2017, 306, 307, 309)

The mother is a frustrating element for the young female homosexual, but the patient doesn't speak to this rejection that Freud notes. Rather, she brings in the lady as a compensatory object. With Dora, the father is the one who brings the lady in the place of the mother. Dora is thus able, straight away, to reproach her father and make known her knowledge of the affair. The personal complaint is much more shrouded in the case of the young female homosexual.

This leaves one case operating, according to Lacan, in the register of the metaphor of the father's love. Dora wonders what her father loves about Frau K. and plays with placing herself in various positions with respect to this love. The other case, Lacan notes, operates through metonymy, a series of equivalent objects that she seeks, the lady being one such object, as is her father's irate gaze. Metaphor grants more of a secured place for the subject. Metonymy leads to a much more dangerous acting-out in the form of a suicidal gesture of throwing herself/falling at the point where she loses the supports she had constructed. Dora's action, on the other hand, was a letter designed to impact the father, but keep herself bound in a constellation of objects.

Freud gets these cases wrong in corresponding inverse form, namely in his position in the transference. Thus, with Dora, he interprets an imaginary element symbolically: he imagines that Dora must recognise her love for Herr K. and her father. With the young female homosexual, he takes what is symbolic and treats it as imaginary: Freud insists that her dreams, which lie about her desire to become heterosexual, is her simply duping him rather than being a symbolic element in and of itself. Lacan writes:

> These two cases balance each other out admirably. They criss-cross, the one with the other, and strictly so, not only because the conflating of the symbolic position and the imaginary position occurs in either case in the opposite direction, but still more because in their overall constellation they are in strict correspondence, with the sole proviso that they are correlated as positive to negative ... [like] perversion is the negative of neurosis.
>
> (Lacan [1956–1957] 2020, 128)

Dora ends her treatment with Freud; Freud ends his treatment with the young female homosexual.

This unpacking of the structure of the two cases by Lacan is moving and elegant. It also functions as a map for listening and depicts a logic inherent to each case. Lacan gives us a model of reading, not only Freud's texts, but where a patient is when they come to treatment, including assessing the potential dangers of acting-out. Love as metaphor is more stabilising than love as metonymic, but it is also more sticky, fixed. The evocation of Dora's question concerning love for women allows her to interrogate and make powerful demands on others. The young female homosexual always stops short of articulating her desire, though she is impressively courageous in her acts. Despite these cases being over one hundred years old, these figures recur constantly in contemporary clinical work.

Dora Even Further Outside

The last time Lacan went into great depth on the Dora case was in his seventeenth seminar, *The Other Side of Psychoanalysis* in 1969–1970. Importantly, this seminar took place in the aftermath of the May 1968 events in Paris. This late reading of Dora acts like a second pass of his "Intervention on Transference" (Lacan [1951] 2006) text, showing the moves in the case, from an outside perspective, through discourse. In this seminar, Lacan inaugurates hysteria as its own discourse making it part of a shared and sharable form, alongside the discourses he names the master, the university, and the analyst. Moving out of discrete structural diagnostics as used in clinical work, by *discourse* Lacan means a way that certain configurations hold together without a subject's speech, providing a position from which to speak.

While one might imagine there are more than simply these four discourses, Lacan says that these are the four that are brought to light by psychoanalysis and are traversed by analyst and analysand. Importantly, between the four there is neither progress nor revolution, just movement. In each discourse we experience the positions from which we speak and produce effects, ones that also entail certain losses. Psychoanalysis creates a new social form, a different way of holding together and speaking, that emerges directly from the hysteric's discourse.

Lacan begins by saying that the hysteric appears in psychoanalysis, often because of a run-in with the master's discourse – the most ancient of discourses where a subject feels equivalent to what they are saying; announcing their rule, power, and sovereignty. Thus, they violate the law, since no one is equal to what they say, and we are, each of us, submitted to the law. The master's discourse takes up an *uncastrated* position of exception to the rule:

In every case, from *Studies in Hysteria* onward, the father is himself made out of symbolic appreciation … And it is in relation to this fact that, in this symbolic field, it must be observed that it is the father, insofar as he plays this pivotal major role, this master role in the hysteric's discourse, that, from this angle of the power of creation, sustains his position in relation to the woman even as he is out of action … it is very precisely this that we designate as the idealized father.
(Lacan [1969–1970] 2007, 95)

We see in the hysteric a question about the master in the form of complaints about enjoyments and privileges, especially in the guise of the father. It is always from the position of the master that the hysteric's place is sustained, even as a sustained struggle.

While she wants to prove that the master is castrated, what the hysteric avoids is a question regarding her *jouissance*. In wielding truth against others, she betrays an unknown enjoyment – perhaps sadistic, perhaps counter-phallic. The hysteric always teaches someone else something precious about the field of the sexual, as Dora did Freud. The precondition of the analyst's discourse is the hysteric's discourse, meaning she creates the possibility of a new discourse around what one does not know, or what cannot enter easily into knowledge. Lacan quips that we often cure everything for a hysteric except her hysteria. How true!

The hysteric's discourse thus defines the position of the analyst as someone who must *not* meet her as a master. "I ask you to refuse what I offer you, because that's not it" is the sentence Lacan kept repeating about himself and hysteria ([1972–1973] 1999, 111). Psychoanalysis, as one of the discourses, produces something new at the place of dissatisfaction and impossibility, or what Lacan calls impotence or powerlessness. Only in this way can the analyst learn something absolutely singular about the hysteric's unconscious life and return this to her.

In the analyst's discourse, knowledge is separated from the important signifiers that emerge in analysis which take place beyond understanding. As analysts we do not act as if we are equal to these signifiers since they come from a place beyond either analyst or analysand. Nor do we see these signifiers as embodied in any given person, idealised or hated (as the hysteric's discourse does). Nor do we saturate an emergent truth with knowledge, especially as etiological explanation (university discourse). What the analyst tries to know more about is how truth emerges from the Other. It is this new kind of knowledge, one Lacan says can be added to the real, that he spends the last decade of his life working on.

The hysteric opens up a question concerning *jouissance* as Other, as an excess, and not simply the filling of a lack. What is repeated in the signifiers that emerge in analysis is the mark of an encounter with the Other as foreign and closed to the subject. A true gap between oneself and the Other. Other *jouissance* is an enigma. The analyst increasingly zeroes in on what *jouissance* reveals in signifiers that mark a subject and insists. "It's from the analyst's discourse that there can emerge another style of master signifier" (Lacan [1969–1970] 2007, 176). This new style of master signifier works with the non-rapport between the sexes, and everything that follows is from Lacan's attention to disjunction, impossibility, and castration. It took the hysteric, and importantly Dora, to echo-locate this liminal terrain.

Twenty-First-Century Doras

I want to present a few cases which will echo the progressive readings of Dora by Lacan, to show how critical hysteria still is to thinking about psychoanalytic work. I worked with a little girl at two points in her life: at age 11 and again when she was 17. She had also been seen as a baby by a psychoanalyst as a rare case of infant anorexia. She had to be fed with a feeding tube for much of her first year and a half of life. The original analyst told me that this was a complicated family with a lot of symptoms exacerbated by the birth of this child which caused them to split up. In working with the family and the toddler, he realised the feeding tube acted as a kind of prop, holding this infant together in a family that was falling apart. They were able to keep the feeding tube in place but begin to feed her regularly. She seemingly progressed well through childhood until she reached her eleventh year when she developed symptoms of anxiety. It was at this point that they brought her to see me. I worked with her for about two years.

What she came to articulate during that time was a point of crisis surrounding her father's break-up with his girlfriend, to whom she had been quite attached. The father had many girlfriends over the years so what was different this time? Well, this girlfriend was friends with the mother, and had verbally attacked the mother during the time the relationship was breaking down for meddling in her relationship. In fact, the mother was often over-involved in her ex-husband's life and love life in one way or another. So, although she wasn't wrong, something had definitely gotten out of hand on both sides. Once the relationship was over, however, the mother revealed the details of her difficulties with this woman to her daughter – in part, I suspect, out of jealousy, since this woman was younger, and my patient enjoyed going to the nail salon with her, going shopping, listening to music, and other activities she didn't share with her mother.

This information from her mother had a powerful retroactive effect. She began to revise her feelings about her relationship with the girlfriend, her idealisation of her came crashing down, bringing to the surface a question about all that she *did not know*. She suddenly felt herself to be in the midst of chaos and violence. She said that she had several anxiety attacks, developed fears of vomiting in public, that began when confronted by bureaucratic tasks having to do with school that normally a parent would handle, but which she often handled because her parents weren't "good at that kind of thing". Up to this crisis point she had been handling all of this, and for quite some time. This begs the question, for whom?

As with infancy, she was propping herself up – through the girlfriend, a certain image of her parents – a scaffolding which fell apart. Anxiety and symptoms erupted. Being able to articulate and pinpoint the moment of confusion and panic eased the anxiety and allowed her to begin to ask some important questions: why did the father have so many relationships and what was his volatility about? Why did the mother lack any relationships? Why did they remain so tied to one another despite separating when she was born? She described different states in her body in their houses. She also described fears about money in this family of artists, and importantly, the mother's depression and the amount she spoke about it to her daughter. Her question was certainly a question about familial *jouissance*, her place in the middle of it. The parents ended treatment because of financial concerns, but I had a feeling that the work was stopped at the place where she might more fully separate herself off from the parental couple. They stopped her separation by stopping the sessions.

I saw her again when she was 17 years old, when she had a similar moment of collapse. She had just left a relationship with a boy that disappointed her greatly, having questions about her bi-sexuality and violence in her culture against people identified as LGBTQ. Depressive feelings arose concerning the way her anxiety constricted her in the same ways she felt it constricted her parents. Importantly, she was finding that the way she had constructed her goals as counter to her parent's lifestyle as impoverished artists, wasn't, in fact, what she wanted. She too wanted to be an artist, and this really alarmed and confused her.

One evening while smoking marijuana, "stressed out" about her life choices, she looked in the mirror and couldn't recognise herself which caused extreme anxiety and she had to go to the emergency room. She subsequently developed severe stomach aches, and continued having feelings that she couldn't recognise her body, that it was out-of-proportion, almost as a kind of return of her infant anorexic symptoms. Once again, this question of *jouissance* tied to her parents, caused the breakdown of certain imagistic constructions that had secured, for a time, a tolerable position for her.

I remember an important session where she had a panic attack just before a break I was taking and our last meeting. She said she wasn't sure why she had it. Recent LGBTQ laws had passed that had upset her, but that didn't seem to explain it. She had a new singing gig, a first paid gig in fact, which was making her nervous – but that still didn't seem enough. She wants to stop sleeping with a boy and she doesn't know if she is with him because she wants to be with him, or wants to be him…

"Hm?" I say.

Then she remembers calling her father just before the panic attack to complain about her job as a waitress and her plan to leave the job, for which he started to berate her.

"Why did you call him?" I asked.

"I don't know. I mean, he complains to me, so why shouldn't I be able to complain to him?"

This led to a fascinating conversation about her being the support of her parents voicing complaints – her mother's depression, her father's worrying and frustration, that she maintained even though it always led in a direction that was as predictable as the upset it caused her.

Her chosen art is singing, an object with the most minimal supports – tied to orality, but existing in relation to it with an important difference. This family seemed to concentrate its *jouissance* around the mouth, a metonymy for the entire body and its passions, difficult to sustain without extreme symptoms bound to one another. What support or position could she find on her own terms? And what could she do with this *jouissance* through the use of her voice?

Another patient, a woman in her thirties, brought fascinating signifiers to bear in her analysis at a critical moment. These began with a dream of babies encased in cement. When listening to the dream I heard "see-meant" which seemed to follow the transference where the patient was constantly testing me to see if she could see what I meant, or, at times, what she meant to me. This took the comical form of asking me what I meant compulsively after every remark, as if I was speaking a foreign language. Less comically, it took the form of suicidal and other threats, especially to the treatment itself. This was a search for something that could cement or encase her, a need for an anchor that was palpable and at times desperate.

The demand in the analysis was intense, as if it was something I could simply provide her with, I suppose, like any demand for love. I felt like she wanted to get me, the analyst, to show her what I mean, linking meaning to the visual register, as if a phonic swerve away from the voice, language, symbolic exchange. Articulation is demanded by the patient in an almost counter-phobic relation to speech, or even, the voice itself; like the texting generation that feels terrorised by voicemail.

There was a period in this analysis when this phobia of the more nonsensical dimension of speech followed the transformation of little Hans' crumpled Giraffe, moving towards this symbolic dimension. I had to be very careful when bringing in the dimension of language which could set off a storm of acting out. Finally, after some very difficult periods, this terrifying voice object in dreams transformed into a letter, written by me to her, or by her to me – this "articulation" she desperately wanted from me and wanted to avoid herself. She said the letter looked like a "bumper sticker". "Bump her … stick her," I said to her. The elements of attachment are a particular emphasis in this patient's analysis, "stick" and "cement", that she adds to the object. Importantly, it should be noted that she hysterically takes the position of the lover (something often thought of as the "masculine position") with respect to me – "stick her" – even as she desires an object from me, to be my beloved.

While the attempt to anchor herself is overwhelmingly present, you begin to see the imaginary object take form as a symbolic circulation, verbal exchange, even the marking that is writing which is there to be read and received as a message. This was a period where she seemed to calm down. She recalled an early memory of feeling desperately confused by her mother's directions, which took the form of not knowing which direction to put her clothes on – how can you know what was the front and what was the back? She would say to her mother "this way, this way" *ad infinitum*, and turn the clothes around and around, as if there was nothing to anchor these signifiers coming from the Other. Indeed, there was something maddening and confusing in the messages that came from this mother. There is also a question about sexual difference embedded in the symptom. She also, at this time, began checking the locks and windows every night before bed.

There was a charming early memory that she linked to some of her current dilemmas around eating. Chicken was one of her favourite foods. She had recently played with a baby chick without quite understanding that it would grow up to be this beloved food. One day at dinner the thought finally occurred to her as she mouthed the word, saying, "chick…chick…chick…chicken!" and promptly started screaming. She refused to eat anything but rice for an entire year, her mother renaming her "rice girl" – but she added that she alarmingly lost a severe amount of weight and had to be taken to the doctor, a kind of prelude for later bouts of anorexia. It isn't just the fact of eating something that you connect with the image of the live animal, it is this discovery as one that takes place through language, the scene unseen, grasping the reality of the adult's *jouissance* through language. A chicken isn't merely the adult chick that is cruelly killed and eaten, a pure object, but also the very image of the adult that can become suddenly grotesque, a display of their impossible enjoyment. The separation between chick and chicken collapses, as does the separation between rice and girl.

How can you *see* what another *means* – as in the colloquial phrase "I see what you mean"? Does this not collapse language and the primal scene? It is true my patient admired a kind of short-hand speech between female best friends where what is said hardly matters aside from maintaining the illusion of mutual, near total, understanding. This tribalist ethos is in fact taking on a life of its own in the United States, a kind of adolescent regressive dream of a world without misunderstanding, meaning, in a way, a world without rotten adults and their rotten sexuality. But the desire for recognition gets the best of them and the dream explodes on the shores of contact or conflict with anyone admired or loved.

In another dream, my patient was given a car by a figure who seemed like the analyst – a "Ford Escape". As she was backing out of the driveway in the midst of an apocalyptic scene, her seat started to move. She immediately jumped out of the car and started screaming, "can someone fix my seat?" and woke up. I wondered with her why she had to stop and ask for help – she hadn't even driven out of the driveway. "My seat was moving," she kept saying over and over, getting increasingly agitated with me as if this was simply obvious. "See moving," I said back to her. She said that seeing this moving was upsetting to her. What will stop this sliding of the signifiers? In another session, she said my office smelled. "Like what?" I asked. "Ceder" … she herself said "see her", she wanted to see me, and then "seed her" to make pregnant, roots.

The hysterical fear of *jouissance* is critical, both sought after and defended against, which brings with it the imagination of feminine and masculine forms of enjoyment: *see her, seed her, see meant, bump her, stick her*. The work of analysis, through work with these signifiers unique to her, was affording her some measure of escape from anxiety, from the experience of life as catastrophic sea changes, and from the compulsive counterstrategy of the attempt to control language through seeking meaning, and dangerous acting out. Both these cases exemplify the oral, acoustic, sexual, and visual dimensions of hysterical symptoms and the logic in which they play out – in life, and then again in psychoanalysis.

Note

1 Lacan departs from Freud's text here, which in fact reads as follows: Herr K. said, "You know I get nothing out of my wife" (Freud 1905, 98).

References

Freud, Sigmund. (1905). "Fragment of an Analysis of a Case of Hysteria". In *The Standard Edition of the Complete Psychological Works of Sigmund Freud*, translated by James Strachey, vol. 7, pp. 1–122. London: Vintage, 1953.

Freud, Sigmund. (1920). "The Psychogenesis of a Case of Homosexuality in a Woman". In *The Standard Edition of the Complete Psychological Works of Sigmund Freud*, translated by James Strachey, vol. 18, pp. 147–172. London: Vintage, 1953.

Freud, Sigmund. (1926). "Inhibitions, Symptoms, and Anxiety". In *The Standard Edition of the Complete Psychological Works of Sigmund Freud*, translated by James Strachey, vol. 20, pp. 77–174, Londo: Vintage, 1953.

Lacan, Jacques. (1951). "Intervention on Transference". In *Écrits: The First Complete Edition in English*, translated by Bruce Fink, pp. 176–185. New York: Norton, 2006.

Lacan, Jacques. (1954–1955). "The Ego in Freud's Theory and in the Technique of Psychoanalysis". In *The Seminar of Jacques Lacan, Book II*, translated by Sylvana Tomaselli, edited by Jacques-Alain Miller. Cambridge: Cambridge University Press, 1988.

Lacan, Jacques. (1955–1956). "The Psychoses". In *The Seminar of Jacques Lacan, Book III*, translated by Russell Grigg, edited by Jacques-Alain Miller. London: W.W. Norton & Co, 1993.

Lacan, Jacques. (1956–1957). "The Object Relation". In *The Seminar of Jacques Lacan, Book IV*, translated by Adrian Price. Cambridge: Polity, 2020.

Lacan, Jacques. (1957–1958). "Formations of the Unconscious". In *The Seminar of Jacques Lacan, Book V*, translated by Russell Grigg. Cambridge: Polity, 2017.

Lacan, Jacques. (1962–1963). "Anxiety". In *The Seminar of Jacques Lacan, Book X*, translated by Adrian Price. Cambridge: Polity, 2014.

Lacan, Jacques. (1969–1970). "The Other Side of Psychoanalysis". In *The Seminar of Jacques Lacan, Book XVII*, translated by Russell Grigg. New York: Norton, 2007.

Lacan, Jacques. (1972–1973). "On Feminine Sexuality, The Limits of Love and Knowledge (Encore)". In *The Seminar of Jacques Lacan, Book XX*, translated by Bruce Fink, edited by Jacques-Alain Miller. New York: Norton, 1999.

YOUNG HOMOSEXUAL WOMAN

Psychogenesis of a Case of Homosexuality in a Woman

MARGARETHE CSONKA

Born 1900, Vienna
Died 1999, Vienna

*One thing I really noticed...
was that "the lady" sounds fantastic!*

Freud, Sigmund. (1920). "Psychogenesis of a Case of
Homosexuality in a Woman". In *The Standard Edition of
the Complete Psychological Works of Sigmund Freud*, translated
by James Strachey, vol. 18, pp. 147–172. London: Hogarth, 1955.

DOI: 10.4324/9781032663746-5

Gender Anxiety as a Symptom of the Analyst

Anouchka Grose

I'm going to presume familiarity with Freud's case of female homosexuality and refer quite tangentially to the things it brought out for me the last time I read it. I'd mainly like to look at the relevance of the case to contemporary clinical practice. Is it just of historical interest? Do you have to read it critically? Is it totally awful in a way that's hard to see if you're a fully indoctrinated Freudian? If I think of some of the 20-year-olds I know reading it, I wonder how they would experience it.

However, the main thing I wanted to look at was the notion of normativity in Freud's case and in some of the Lacanian thinking around gender and sexuality. Freud is pretty upfront and unapologetic about it when he says: "In general, to undertake to convert a fully developed homosexual into a heterosexual does not offer much more prospect of success than the reverse, except that for good practical reasons the latter is never attempted" (Freud 1920, 151).

Maybe it's all part of being a Freud apologist – we always tend to see what's radical and exciting in his thinking and sometimes forget to take seriously the aspects of it that are more normative. It's as if the *good* bits are the printed words and the *bad* bits are the blank page. But maybe the page is as important as the words; no paper, no words. On the bright side, he's clearly saying that curing homosexuality is a bad idea; it's not going to work, so don't bother. And it would have been great if certain of his followers had taken that seriously. But he's also saying it stands to reason that no one in their right mind would choose to be homosexual because it puts you at odds with the dominant culture – and why would a person opt to be disadvantaged in that way? So he's simultaneously defending a person's right to have a same-sex partner because that's actually a perfectly regular, unsurprising outcome of the Oedipus complex, while at the same time basically upholding the system that makes having a same-sex partner extremely difficult because…well… that's just the way it is.

It's often presented as a core tenet of Lacanian clinical work that we are anti-normative – that we can't know in advance what's best for our patients, that we have to listen out for the particularities of each case. And also that one's gender position and object choices are arrived at as a result of complex processes and are subject to a huge amount of variability and fluidity. Just because you find something that works for a while, it doesn't follow that it will work forever, and so on. So the great

DOI: 10.4324/9781032663746-6

advantage for me of Lacanian theory over – say – object relations theory, is that you completely let go of *any* idea of knowing what's best for people. You have no notion of a *good object relation* for a start. In fact, that's pretty much the only reason I would identify as a Lacanian. I'm not exactly in love with the theory, nor with the figure of Lacan himself, and can't stand the way it positions itself as superior to all other theories, especially other psychoanalytic orientations. But I do think anti-normativity is a very important thing to bear in mind in clinical practice – we're not there to help people fit in better. So I get peeved about those places where normativity creeps into Lacanian discourse because anti-normativity is the pay-off for putting up with all the *theory bros* and jargon. For instance, in the Lacanian world, it's still absolutely commonplace to hear people reiterate Catherine Millot's (1990) idea from *Horsexe* that trans people are necessarily psychotic because gender isn't a question for them. Or because it's a question that's been answered with a high level of certainty.

Thankfully that's been counter-balanced by people like Patricia Gherovici who've taken the time to look at what Lacan actually does and doesn't say. And, of course, the point isn't to find out what Lacan actually said, as if that's inherently better than what other people might say, but to use certain of his ideas to think further – which a book like Gherovici's *Please Select Your Gender* (2010) does. It might sound funny – or dreadful – to people outside our bubble, but from inside we might understand that it is a very important theoretical recalibration to point out that trans people might just as well be neurotic as psychotic. It's hardly an idea that's going to go well for anyone on Twitter (now known as X), but for people who don't see neurosis and psychosis as illnesses or pathologies but as structures, it's just another way of saying that you can't leap to conclusions about trans people any more than you can about cisgendered people; assumptions will just get in the way of listening.

So what's this got to do with Freud's case? At first glance it looks like an outlandishly antique case – who would send their kid to a psychoanalyst to get them straightened out? In many parts of the world, it's actually illegal. Having said that, I have a friend who practises in another part of the world and it's good to be reminded that different cultures produce different symptoms. He has a clinic full of people who are worried they might be gay, or whose parents are worried they might be gay, or who have a same-sex partner but keep it secret, or a beardy marriage, and so on.

However, the thing he doesn't see in his clinic, or his life, and which is a very prominent part of my work – and my life – is non-binary people. I also noticed just in the last week or two that when speaking to colleagues about it, I'd hear things back that made it clear that psychoanalysts were in totally different places on that subject – like thinking the term *non-binary* was another way of saying *bisexual*. One eminent Lacanian even asked whether I thought it was a cover for being bisexual, and another person just said, "Oh dear." Freud's list of three sets of variables at the end of his case: physical sexual characteristics, mental sexual characteristics, and object choice (Freud 1920, 170) don't seem to have landed with all psychoanalysts. They don't all grasp that your biology, your gender identifications, and your object choice aren't in any kind of inevitable, generic relation to one another; they don't follow Freud in understanding that knowing someone identified as non-binary would in no way tell you anything about their object choice.

Of course, what people say in public and what people say in private may be totally different things, but if that's what a number of my colleagues are saying to me in private, then it made me curious. Why are some psychoanalysts so un-Freudian when they're having dinner?

Then again, there's Patricia Gherovici's (2010) excellently helpful formulation that *the psychoanalytic subject emerges when identity fails*. If you cling rigidly to any identity, it's bound to alienate you. You can discuss this a bit further in terms of diagnosis – identifications may be very helpful for stabilising psychoses; undermining people's identities and identifications certainly isn't what you'll be aiming for in all clinical work. But we can probably loosely agree that the mirror phase doesn't land you anywhere you particularly want to be – it's a recipe for frustration and disappointment. Therefore, fixations on various gender identities might be unhelpful to people and, as psychoanalysts, we might see it as our job to help them put that sort of thing in question. But maybe sometimes, for some practitioners, that seems to translate into the idea that we should be putting *some* people's gender identifications into question and not others. As if identifying as non-binary, say, was necessarily an off-the-peg and therefore suspect solution – something to interrogate and maybe coax your patient away from. In other words, following Freud in thinking it's best for people to follow the path of least resistance. However, if someone turns up and identifies as a straight, cisgendered woman, would you immediately see it as your job to help them put *that* in question? Would you only do so if they happened to put it in question themselves? You'd leave it up to them to question it or not. And would you also only question a trans man or woman, or non-binary person, about their gender position if they brought up the question themselves? Would you think they were psychotic if they didn't bring up the question? Would you think the cis-het woman was psychotic if she didn't want to interrogate her gender identity and object choice? Maybe you would. Maybe you should. Maybe that's exactly a place where you can spot what kind of structure you're dealing with. But that isn't what's being said in some of the Lacanian literature on the subject. It's a bit like the question of punctuality in other orientations – being early or late tends to be interpreted, but never being on time. Why not? Some people's hyper-punctuality is quite notable and surely says as much about them as fluctuations around timing in either direction.

In Genevieve Morel's book, *Sexual Ambiguities*, which came out in 2011, a year after *Please Select Your Gender*, she writes:

> In the psychoanalytic clinic of the neuroses, it is extremely rare to find an individual who has such absolute certainty about his/her sex. They may ask, "Am I a real woman? Aren't I too masculine?" or "Am I really masculine? Aren't I too weak to be a man?", etc. The subject has doubts and worries about traits that

may indicate the presence of the other sex in him/herself. Sometimes it takes an entire analysis to sort this problem out. Indeed Lacan characterised neurosis as a question, and hysteria in particular as a question about sex: "Am I a man or a woman?" On the other hand, a subject who attributes such certainty to his/her sex that he/she is prepared to submit to surgery, may well be psychotic, even if he/she appears perfectly normal.

(Morel 2011, 59)

You could say, "Oh, well, Morel is just talking about different types of people" – but she does use the word *normal* in that last sentence. Surgery is set up here as a diagnostic indicator of psychosis and therefore non-normality, which is not at all the same as saying everyone's unique and particular. She also suggests that uncertainty around gender is a problem that might be sorted out in analysis. Of course, you could say you'll never sort it out, but at least analysis might help you to suffer the uncertainty a little less. This would seem a great thing to say, but this is not what Morel is saying or at least included in what she's setting up as a binary between normal and not normal, where trans people are on the wrong side.

*****

Another thing I noticed about Freud's case with the young homosexual girl was that he seemed to feel very free to interrogate cause and effect, and to attribute the phenomena of this woman's sexual and romantic life to conscious and unconscious reactions to things that were happening in her family. "She's running around after a woman because her sexy, rivalrous mum had a baby", and so on. The girl's homosexuality is being treated like a symptom, even if it's a symptom Freud has no intention of curing. Her homosexuality is a solution to a set of problems she's run into, which you could also presumably say about any other object choice. But the thing that struck me about it – although on the surface it's what you do in psychoanalysis, you look into cause and effect – is that the way you come at those questions in the consulting room is very important.

   About ten years ago, an analysand of mine went to a psychoanalytic institute to be interviewed for the training. When he told his interviewer he was gay, she said, "So what went wrong then?" He'd previously had the idea that the Institute was where all the proper psychoanalysts hung out and that he was slumming it with me, so he was absolutely amazed and horrified to discover that such a question could be asked in such a way. He decided to stick with being an artist. It's so outlandish, it seems like a caricature, but I have sometimes felt pushed towards the role of that kind of analyst by one of my non-binary analysands who used to say things to me like, "I'm just waiting for you to say something stupid and then I won't be able to speak to you anymore." Nothing makes it more likely that you will say something stupid than someone saying that to you. Still, maybe part of being a cisgendered white person is that you have to suck up that risk and that worry. It comes with the privilege – it's what you pay. It also seemed as though there might be even worse things than the possibility of directly misgendering this person or referring to them as their mum's daughter, or some other bit of linguistic clumsiness. If there was going to be a problem, it probably wouldn't be that. The risk seemed more that I might try to open up the possibility of thinking that there were things in their life that had led them to that particular gender identification, and that this in itself would be an affront. Any suggestion of cause and effect risked seeming pathologising, so I just had to accept that certain things about this person "just were", but that everything else was up for discussion. I'm sure any dyed-in-the-wool Lacanian would therefore leap to the conclusion that this person is psychotic – taking as further proof the fact that they don't appear psychotic in the slightest, and that there are plenty of neurotic phenomena there just to throw you off the trail. But I can't see any good reason to leap to that conclusion. Maybe some neurotic people are excellent at shutting down certain avenues for discussion, and maybe in time this person will become curious about certain very striking aspects of their biography that maybe do have a bearing on how they experience gender. Maybe the question isn't so much neurosis or psychosis, but time and trust.

So, for Freud, in the case of the homosexual girl, perhaps one striking thing is his evident freedom to ask, "Why is this person like this?" And to answer purely in terms of their mum, their dad, their brother, their desires and identifications inside the family. And of course we can't know from his write-up of the case how much of this was being interpreted back to the patient, and how much was just being observed. You might very well ask those same sorts of questions in a contemporary case but perhaps with a different emphasis. So in Freud, in spite of all the great things he has to say about not attempting to cure homosexuality, the drive behind the questions seems to be to work out why this girl has chosen this woman as her love object.

One thing I really noticed this time when reading the case was that "the lady" sounds fantastic. She certainly embodies a kind of contemporary ideal – her sexuality seems very fluid. She's in a relationship with a woman but she sees men. She's a blue-chip sex worker. She's the kind of cool, emancipated person you get after the various waves of sexual revolution helped along by psychoanalysis. She lives ethically outside societal norms – she wants what's best for Sidonie, Freud's patient. All of which is to say it's funny that Freud is so hard at work asking. "Why, why, why does Sidonie fancy this woman?" when for many of us it might seem pretty self-evident.

When there's a cautiousness around one's mode of questioning in analytic work – or maybe a watchfulness around your mode of questioning by an analysand – it's good to remember that it isn't questions *per se* that are the problem, but where you place the emphasis, or what you seem to be going after. So with the person who keeps such a close eye on me in the work we do together, it seems helpful to me to remember that the question isn't *what makes you non-binary?* but *what makes you unhappy?* And maybe if we keep the emphasis there, we will eventually open up questions around the things that need to be spoken about – when the time's right for the person to look at those things, if that's what they want to do. Perhaps you have to create the conditions for those questions to become interesting or bearable, rather than saying, "That person doesn't have questions about their gender, therefore they're psychotic."

This is a very generalising thing to say, but I do wonder sometimes with the things I hear from colleagues whether there isn't often a kind of anxiety or paranoia about the idea that you're just supporting *the discourse* – you're being pushed around by the culture and your freedom to think is being limited. But why? This certainly isn't restricted to gender or sexuality. I was amazed in a recent seminar when a colleague said he couldn't understand why psychoanalysts seemed so reluctant to question the science around climate change when we question the science in other areas of life. For example, the science of psychiatric medication is under constant bombardment by members of our profession. If you have the idea that psychoanalysts are meant to put received wisdom in question that's one thing, but surely being a flat-earther is something else...

One very clear place you can see this idea of pandering to the discourse is in Jacques Alain Miller's response to Paul Preciado in a text titled "Docile de Trans" (Miller 2020), which is all about not letting yourself be pushed around by pesky trans people and their supposedly misguided allies. I'm not on Twitter so I don't know the blow-by-blow stuff that goes on but I've read Paul Preciado's (2021) book, *Can the Monster Speak?* which I liked and found interesting – he has a brilliant, flashy literary style – and Miller's response to it which made my skin crawl from the everyday sexism on the first page – he refers to a journalist as a "pretty young mother" apropos of nothing – to the cringey way he describes Lacan "giving him the hand" of his most beautiful daughter (and making a passing comment about her power to castrate) before going on to make haughty comments about his sucker of a grandson for speaking about his transfeminine school-friend in the way in which the school-friend wishes to be spoken about.

The Morel book is more nuanced – although it's strange to read a whole book attacking Judith Butler's work that doesn't once mention Judith Butler. The idea of gender as purely performative appears there as either a naïve or a psychotic notion. Neurotics, we are told, accept the Name-of-the-Father and are therefore submitted to the phallic function. They may not like the idea of binaries, nor the castrating aspect of accepting one's assigned gender, but they can deal with it in a begrudging, neurotic way. They want to find ways around it, and they do find all sorts of perverse, twisted ways to make a bit of a mess of it but, in the end, they can see where the limits lie and work around them or complain about them – but basically accommodate them because – well – what else are you going to do? Psychotic people, however, don't have phallic law to keep things in place so have to make up *crazy* systems and principles of their own. Here's a quote from Morel, from the same book:

> In a certain way, it [the concept of transsexualism] is a psychotic concept. This concept takes as "the truth" of sex what is in fact an "elementary phenomenon" of transsexualism: the delusional conviction that there has been an error of nature in determining the subject's sex. In a certain way.
>
> (Morel 2011, 59)

In this quote she's alluding to the work of Robert Stoller from 1968 in his influential book *Sex and Gender*, where he coins the term *gender identity* and puts the trans experience down to faulty imprinting caused by faulty mothering. I'll just give you a bit more of the Morel book to show how strongly she drives home her point about trans people and psychosis:

> In psychosis … the Name of the Father is foreclosed, and the subject is delivered up to the mother's whim without the mediation of the paternal law. It is not surprising then that transsexuals have been their mother's privileged object, an *object a*, and that they are feminized, either by an early and massive identification with the mother, or because they have been subject to a *pousse-à-la-femme*. This is where there is a psychotic feminization forced upon the subject, whether the latter is anatomically a man or a woman.
>
> (Morel 2011, 60)

To come back to the contemporary clinic, to me, this would suggest a certain level of disengagement from what goes on in the lives of actual trans people. First of all, generic trans narratives about living in the wrong body are pretty much no longer a thing. Maybe they were in 1968 but that may very often have been because that's what trans people thought they had to say in order to be taken seriously. In particular, "I was born in the wrong body" is precisely *not* what you hear from anyone these days, perhaps because there are far more spaces (both physical and online) where trans people can have thoughtful conversations and compare experiences with other trans people. The phrase is an echo from the days when you just had to reach for something standard issue in order to get your point across to an uncomprehending listener. But the problem with this outdated myth is that it sets up a standard for what a *real* trans person should be like.

What you do hear in the contemporary clinic is how varying degrees of certainty and uncertainty about your gender can really complicate things for you when you go to a clinic in order to start discussing the possibility of surgery or hormones. For many people, if they show any hint of self-questioning or doubt, they'll be told to go away and come back in a year, having given the matter further thought or maybe done some therapy. And this is just to get a psychiatric letter of support to apply for private treatment, which involves a whole other layer of vetting. Because the discourse around trans has moved along so much elsewhere, people might turn up to these clinics imagining the discourse will have moved on in the clinics too. So they might speak honestly to the people doing the assessments, trying to give truthful, nuanced answers, and then find themselves being knocked back and told to make another appointment in a year's time to see whether they're any more sure about what they want.

Over and over again what I hear in my practice is people speaking interestingly and in subtle, complex ways, or maybe they speak with friends, or in their writing, but then if they want to get the official go-ahead, they have to put all their careful thinking to one side and just be very definite and unequivocal. In other words, they have to play dumb in order to work a system that cannot handle their subjectivity but can only work with crass identifications and identities. Anything else just makes the people operating the system too nervous.

You might say, well, it's good that the gatekeepers of hormones and surgery are nervous types because it's not good to be offering people permanent changes to their bodies and reproductive systems that they might regret later, etc., etc. But I think you see in the quotes from the Morel book that people can sometimes be very jumpy about body modifications, as if they're something quite beyond the pale. But maybe *that* is a thing that could be questioned, if questioning things is some kind of sovereign good. When does body modification come to indicate a psychosis? Only when it has to do with gender? What about breast enlargements? Facelifts? Could go either way! It's OK as long as it's a good, natural-looking facelift? Are tattoos suspect? It almost seems funny, but it isn't funny if clinicians who live quite sheltered lives are making judgements about their patients and trying to move them towards various kinds of conformity because that's what seems to work for the clinicians themselves. And this really isn't what we see Freud doing in his case. It seems more that he has some standard, commonsensical opinions but, as far as we can tell, he doesn't explicitly impose these on the patient.

In *Testo Junkie*, Paul Preciado (2008) argues that developments in medicine open up all sorts of possibilities around what you have to accept and what you don't. If you get cancer you don't necessarily have to accept death. But also, if you can't get an erection, you can take Viagra. Or you can use the pill to avoid pregnancy. You can have your hormones rebalanced. You don't have to accept menopause in quite the same way. Medicine doesn't treat the body as sealing the fate of the subject. There are all sorts of things you can do if you want to dodge the fate either coded into your body or set out in the meeting of body and world. One argument of Preciado's book is that once you have the pharmaceutical terrain that we currently have, you necessarily also have the capacity to do more sophisticated things with gender. Once you have the pill, HRT and Viagra, you're going to get all the rest. In his book, he describes his use of testosterone to move towards a masculine position and describes how it's tied in with an affair he's having with a woman; the excitement of the affair and the excitement of hormonal changes elide with each other.

In a later book, *Can the Monster Speak*, Preciado (2021) speaks about his transition, which didn't involve surgery at all, only the use of hormones. He describes the satisfaction that comes with passing as a man, but also points out that, in his case, it's perfectly reversible. And that's certainly something that happens often enough; you see people go through it in analysis and it's fine. This whole business of equating surgery with gender transitioning and using the idea of the irreversibility of surgery as an indicator of something extreme, unquestioning, and therefore psychotic isn't commensurate with the contemporary state of gender reassignment, either medically or culturally.

In fact, if people want to talk about certainty and uncertainty and to make diagnostic points about it, the certainty that gender is binary and civilisation and law will collapse if we ignore that hard-coded reality can start to seem like the *madder* position. For example, Nina Power's (2022) recent book sets out with the idea that, "All human life stems from the reality of, and difference between, men and women." It's a book which is ostensibly psychoanalytic or at least its title is: *What Do Men Want?: Masculinity and its Discontents*. It's full of the idea that if we lose the father, we will all suffer because of the loss of protection and also the loss of an organising principle. Lacan is also an adherent of this idea, for instance, it appears in the "Family Complexes" ([1938] 2003) essay. But the problem, at least in the Nina Power book, is that the perversity that can be enacted through the *caring* masculine role is completely ignored in favour of the idea that men may be straightforwardly *nice*. Power argues, for example, that above all she wants *to defend the possibility today of connecting masculinity to goodness.*

Karen Barad (2007), who works with feminist and queer theory, combining it with physics, has what seems to me a useful way of thinking about the so-called *real* of gender. You can think of it in terms of Newtonian physics and quantum physics. It's true to say that the laws of classical mechanics are demonstrably operative on Earth. Things behave in certain ways that are explicable by a certain set of formulations. That's all *real*. We have gravity and air resistance, and Newton obviously came up with some very functional ways of thinking about all that. But once you leave the very particular conditions of our planet and start thinking about the universe, those equations break down. Time and space are no longer calculable in the same ways. Things bend and fold, and sequentiality doesn't necessarily hold up in the ways we might expect. So there's one set of rules governing the surface of our planet, and another set of rules governing the universe that surrounds our planet. One exists inside the other. And those two sets of rules are in relation, but sometimes they may be at odds. You certainly can't extrapolate outwards from Earth to space in any simple way; the sensible, explicable things we have going on around us are not at all the same as the difficult-to-think but equally *real* stuff happening beyond our perception and comprehension. So maybe using 1960s medicine and gender theory as your reference point for how gender might be thought or experienced now is like using classical mechanics to talk about what goes on in space. You can say, "Grrr, Newton's right, it's a demonstrably true, rational theory, anyone who argues with it is crazy", and that might be right if all you're thinking about is what goes on in your immediate locale, but if you start thinking beyond your locale you might see things start to warp and become a lot more complex and interesting.

So we have to make a distinction between the idea of sexuation, and then performative theories of gender, and something like the hard-coded but also quasi-mystical/natural notions of gender in the Nina Power book, as perhaps these latter are the most overtly *Newtonian*. You might even want to argue that Lacan's theory of sexuation is just the quantum idea we need. The problem is that it gets used to support ideas about transitioning and gender fluidity that seem to align better with a more straightforwardly anti-trans stance – the stance that says, "it's OK to play – we're cool, we love all that, just don't do anything *real* to your body and don't bring the law or language into it otherwise we're all doomed." You get all these points of allegiance and of difference between the theories that can be quite hard to untangle.

Just to give a quick, schematic account of sexuation, it follows a kind of sequential logic. Initially you have the biological difference between men and women, then you have the discourse around sex and gender – which would tend to mean the discourse inside the family, rather than *the discourse* at large, and may be the kind of discourse that simply backs up biology, or it might not – that depends on your family, and finally *a choice* that the subject has to make about where they position themselves with regard to all that. So sexuation is apparently a subtle theory and better than all other theories of gender – *haha!* – because it invokes subjectivity. So that's great, gender is a big headfuck and it's unstable and completely idiosyncratic in each case – *blah, blah, blah!* But then you get ideas like this one from the Morel book again, from the section where she discusses sexuation. She's talking about Lacan's idea of the "common error" regarding the phallus. That basically we all misunderstand the place it has for us, but this misunderstanding somehow binds us together in communities of mistakenness. So here's the quote: "The term 'error' here is a nod towards transsexuals and their discourse, which exposes 'the error of nature' of which they are the victims: they have not been born into the 'right' sex" (Morel 2011, 132).

Even when someone is outlining this supposedly subtle theory regarding everyone's precious particularity, you get the idea of transsexuals being lumped together under one narrative as if all trans people experience gender in the same way.

I've noticed a kind of terror around talking about this stuff. I know that at our training organisation plenty of people seem to have the idea that we mustn't talk about it because if we do, we can only fall on one side or other of a dividing line where both sides are bad. Either you get into trouble for being *anti-trans* or for being non-Lacanian. And to some Lacanians, that's scary. There's the idea that you have to parrot the discourse or risk cancellation, but this notion of an angry trans person who will cancel you is in itself transphobic.

I think all this anxiety around gender and identity gives some people a problem in their clinical work. If the analyst accepts the subject's stated position, are they just being a sucker to the discourse? Are they letting that person's identity alienate them from their subjectivity? Isn't it our job to undo that? But what do you lose by listening to trans people and learning from them rather than coming at them with a set of fully sewn-up terms?

I know it's mostly adherents to other analytic orientations who worry about *colluding with the patient*, as if that's the worst analytic crime. If you're not putting them in question over everything they say and do, then what are you for? This is the whole *why are you late?* thing… But the Jacques-Alain Miller idea of *docility* to trans seems to echo this rather paranoiac attitude: isn't the culture getting one over on you? Shouldn't you be resisting? And so on.

To conclude, I suppose I just wanted to bring out something that can feel like a deadlock between psychoanalysis and *the discourse*, as if the discourse dictates that you're not supposed to ask questions any longer, and we *must* ask questions.

So to finish. This can maybe bring us back to Freud's case and the charming idea that it was once safe to ask questions, because maybe at the time no one was going to question your questions – or at least if they did, they were going to be coming at you from the side of convention and tradition. But perhaps, for whatever reason, some psychoanalysts don't mind being seen as dangerous radicals and revolutionaries, but they get really stressed out when anyone suggests they are being hopelessly normative.

References

Barad, Karen. (2007). *Meeting the Universe Halfway: Quantum Physics and the Entanglement of Matter and Meaning*. Durham, NC: Duke University Press.

Freud, Sigmund. (1920). "Psychogenesis of a Case of Homosexuality in a Woman". In *The Standard Edition of the Complete Psychological Works of Sigmund Freud*, edited by James Strachey, vol. 18, pp. 147–172. London: Hogarth, 1955.

Gherovici. Patricia. (2010). *Please Select Your Gender: From the Invention of Hysteria to the Democratizing of Transgenderism*. New York: Routledge.

Lacan, Jacques. (1938). "Family Complexes in the Formation of the Individual", translated by Cormac Gallagher. London: Karnac Books. 2003.

Miller, Jacques-Alain. (2020). "Docile de Trans". Available at: https://www.lacan.com/pdfjam2021.pdf.

Millot, Catherine. (1990). *Horsexe: Essays on Transsexuality*. New York: Autonomedia.

Morel, Genevieve. (2011). *Sexual Ambiguities*. New York: Routledge.

Power, Nina. (2022). *What Do Men Want?: Masculinity and Its Discontents*. Milton Keynes: Allen Lane.

Preciado, Paul. (2008). *Testo Junkie: Sex, Drugs and Biopolitics in the Pharmacopornographic Era*. New York: The Feminist Press at the City University of New York.

Preciado, Paul. (2021). *Can the Monster Speak? A Report to an Academy of Psychoanalysts*. London: Fitzcarraldo Editions.

Stoller. Robert. (1968). *Sex and Gender: The Development of Masculinity and Femininity*. New York: Routledge.

Chapter 4

Girl, Interrupted

Patricia Gherovici

Why would Freud (1920) take into treatment a girl "who was in no way neurotic" (p. 158, n. 2), whom he admitted "was not in any way ill (she did not suffer from anything in herself, nor did she complain of her condition)" (p. 150)?[1] Nevertheless, at some time between 1918 and 1919, Freud treated Margarethe Csonka (Gretl Trautenegg), a vibrant 18-year-old hailing from an affluent Viennese family, who entered analysis under the watchful eye of her father following an infatuation with an older woman that sparked a scandal, and culminated in a suicide attempt.[2] Amidst such adverse conditions, Freud acknowledged the challenging terrain for psychoanalytic intervention and refrained from offering false assurances to her parents.

Freud was mindful of the limitations and potentials of psychoanalytic practice in such tricky circumstances. Recognising homosexuality not as a pathology but as a variant of human sexuality equally as contingent as heterosexuality, Freud approached the situation with discernment, understanding that psychoanalysis wasn't positioned to *cure* homosexuality or enforce adaptation to prevailing social mandates.[3] In October 1920, Freud, grappling with his unease over the case, wrote to Edoardo Weiss outlining scenarios wherein psychoanalytic intervention might not be advisable. Freud highlighted instances devoid of "painful conflict" or where a patient's distress stemmed primarily from external circumstances rather than internal struggle (Freud and Weiss 1975, 49). Indeed, Margarethe's case epitomised what Weiss (1970) termed the absence of "conflict of suffering". Freud noted that since Gretl lacked any neurotic tendencies and presented not even a single hysterical symptom (Freud 1920, 155), his task therefore had to be nuanced, pivoting neither on the resolution of neurotic strife nor on the transformation of one configuration of genital sexuality into another (pp. 150–151). Taking distance from the social norms of his time, Freud argued that homosexuality was as much an outcome of the Oedipus complex as heterosexuality and equally baffling. He noted, not without irony that, "to undertake to convert a fully developed homosexual into a heterosexual does not offer much more prospect of success than the reverse" (p. 151).

While the girl presented no symptom, her intimate relationship with a baroness who "in spite of her distinguished name" was "nothing but a *cocotte*" (p. 147; italics in the original) had sparked disarray in the Csonka family. The father disapproved

DOI: 10.4324/9781032663746-7

of his daughter's affection for the lady and tried to stop the relationship. Defying the prohibitions, Margarethe continued courting the ill-reputed lady until the day when her father ran into them on the street. He threw a furious glance at the pair before proceeding on his way. The young woman confessed that the irate man was her own father, who had forbidden their friendship. Incensed, the lady stated that under those circumstances she did not wish to see her ever again. On hearing those words, Gretl rushed to the overpass of a railway line nearby and jumped. She was badly injured in this serious attempt at suicide even though in the end she survived with little permanent damage – she nevertheless had to spend months on her back recovering.

Freud noticed the verb that Margarethe used to describe her fall had been *niederkommen*, meaning both "to fall" and "to deliver a child". Freud linked this to a moment in her adolescence when her Oedipus complex had been revived, that is, that she had wished to have her father's child when her mother gave birth to a younger brother. Even though she unconsciously hated her mother for this, she then turned to her, renouncing her womanhood, and having "changed into a man", for a while took her mother in place of her father as a love object, thus overcompensating for the hostility she had felt for her mother. This is a phenomenon that Lacan ([1956–1957] 1994) called a "reactional phenomenon" (p. 98).

Freud noted a curious discrepancy in the parents' attitudes regarding their daughter's homosexuality: the father was furious and unforgiving while the mother tacitly approved. The mother's tolerance was an implicit appreciation of the secret meaning of her daughter's choice – Margarethe's obvious lack of interest in men was a way of avoiding rivalry between daughter and mother since the latter was still a youngish woman who cherished male attention. On his side, the father was quite embittered because of his daughter's defiance. Her turning away from men altogether meant that she was turning away from him as well.

All in all, Lacan followed Freud's analysis of the attempted suicide as having represented both a punishment and a wish fulfilment – "the wish to have a child by her father, for now she 'fell' through her father's fault" (Freud 1920, 162). Margarethe's desperate gesture contained the ultimate and original meaning of the situation (Lacan [1956–1957] 1994, 94–98). Her fall on the railway was a symbolic act according to Freud, it was the *Niederkommen* (delivery) of a baby during childbirth.

Notably, Lacan's discussion of the case focused neither on hysteria nor on homosexuality but on female sexuality, specifically on the disadvantages in which women find themselves when they access their own sexual identity. In an earlier seminar, Lacan argued that this disadvantage was "turned to her advantage in hysteria owing to her imaginary identification with the father, who is perfectly accessible to her, particularly by virtue of his position in the composition of the Oedipus complex" ([1955–1956] 1993, 172). Lacan compared Margarethe to Dora, two women who loved a woman like a man, following what Freud described as "manly type" (*männliches Typus*) to address a question to a woman. In both cases, there was a father, a daughter, and an older woman. As with Dora, the object that Margarethe desired was located beyond the woman she worshipped. For Margarethe, her fervent love was close to the devoted adoration of courtly love. It was an impossible love that took as object what the loved woman was lacking. Lacan concluded that in the extremity of her passionate love, what she looked for in the loved woman was the phallus.

It is clear that Dora's and Margarethe's cases were determined by a whole economy, and that they followed a circuit of gift exchanges (Lacan [1956–1957] 1994, 132). For both, the fathers' inability to give the phallus yielded a new twist to the idea of giving. Dora remained attached to a father whose virile gift she could not receive. Yet, she loved her deficient father all the more, her love growing stronger in inverse proportion to his diminished status (Lacan [1962–1963] 2014, 109). Similarly, Margarethe loved the lady with total devotion and expected nothing in return. She wanted above all to demonstrate to her father that true love is disinterested, which corresponds rather neatly to Lacan's notion that the true sign of love is to give what one does not have (p. 108). Margarethe had wanted to show to her father that one could love someone not for what this person *has* but rather for what the person literally *does not have*.

Lacan's reading of the cases is underpinned by a system of exchanges influenced by Lévi-Strauss's structural anthropology, in which the basic rule of kinship and exogamic exchanges is summed up in the formula "I have received a wife and I owe a daughter" (Lacan [1956–1957] 1994, 136). This principle transforms any woman into an object of exchange. In the social exchange, the male is reduced to being the holder of the phallus. It is the dissymmetry in the phallic function that creates the opposition summed up by Freud as "having" and "not having", a couple that becomes for Lacan a starker opposition between "having" and "being" (Lacan [1962–1963] 2014, 108). Man "has" the phallus, while woman does not have it. Because of that, she can embody it, and thus "be" the phallus (p. 109).

In all this, the function of the father in the mother's discourse has a decisive role to play since hysterics are sustained by their love for the father, even when they deny it. Indeed, the love for the father played a decisive role in Margarethe's attempted suicides. The biography by Ines Rieder and Diana Voigt mentions two other attempts, one with poison, the other with a gun, both having the father as main addressee. In 1922, Margarethe, rejected, hopeless, and disappointed in the lady, feeling trapped after consenting to be courted by a male suitor just to please her father, drank poison (Rieder and Voigt 2019, 104–106).

The third attempt against her life was in 1924. Margarethe was engaged and about to get married. The white bridal dress was already ordered, the reception was scheduled, and the honeymoon plans with visits to Venice and Florence were advancing. But she panicked at the idea of life with a man. Desperate, through the father of a friend, an arms collector, she bought a revolver under the excuse that it was a wedding gift for her fiancé. Margarethe's reason to commit suicide was that she was "afraid to tell her father the truth" about her misgivings about the wedding (p. 129). Not long after a lush engagement party, at night, while all the family was at home sleeping, she took the gun and, aiming at her chest, pulled the trigger. Everyone heard the shot and ran to her help. Margarethe survived because her father promptly took her to the hospital: "Papsel's [daddy] big Steyer-Coupe" madly sped through the streets carrying Sido, groaning in pain, on the back seat (p. 156). Incredibly, the bullet missed her heart by half an inch.

A few months earlier, in August 1924, Margarethe had decided to finally end her relationship with the baroness. The way she chose to break up reveals the crucial role played by her father in her love affair. Margarethe sent her a telegram. "REQUEST YOU CEASE ALL CONTACT WITH MY DAUGHTER. ANTAL CSILLAG" (p. 122). The text was hers, but she signed it with her father's name – Margarethe's love for her father found its expression in revenge against the lady. Margarethe defied the father's desire while trying unsuccessfully to sustain it.

Margarethe gives a twist to the formula "hysteric's desire is desire of/for desire", because, as Lacan ([1964] 1998) observes,

> the formula that originated in the experience in the hysteric—*[hu]man's desire is the desire of the Other*—it is in the desire of the father that the female homosexual finds another solution, that is to defy the desire of the father.
>
> (p. 38; italics in the original)

The father is also at the centre in the interruptions of both Margarethe's and Dora's analyses. Like Dora, and for similar reasons, Margarethe never completed her analysis. Agnès Aflalo-Lebovits (1984) pointed out that after ending his work with Margarethe, Freud revisited Dora's case and assessed in a different light the precipitating factors for Dora's decision to leave the treatment (p. 23).

Freud's Blind Spot

For Dora, in Lacan's commentary, what Freud missed was the fundamental "question on the subject of her sex" ([1955–1956] 1993, 171). This derived from a more general principle:

> for the girl as much as for the boy the castration complex assumes a pivotal value in bringing about the Oedipus complex; it does so precisely as a function of the father, because the phallus is a symbol to which there is no correspondent, no equivalent. It is a matter of dissymmetry in the signifier.
>
> ([1955–1956] 1993, 176)

The symbolic register, which defines the main structure of the link of the unconscious with kinship, lacks a corresponding female equivalent to the phallus. Following Lacan's analysis of how the phallus operates for Dora and Margarethe, we see that the phallus cannot be reduced to an anatomical organ. Lacan talked about the phallus as symbolic object ([1956–1957] 1994, 145) and as a signifier (p. 183). The idea that the phallus should function as a signifier was taken up again in *Seminar V* (Lacan [1957–1958] 2017) and became a central element in the formulation that "the phallus is the signifier of the Other's desire" (Lacan [1958b] 2006, 583).

What was Lacan trying to illustrate with this idea? In his theoretical itinerary, the phallus played an essential role as signifier of sexual difference. Initially, Lacan had distinguished the phallus from the penis, when this phallus was first and foremost an image. The imaginary phallus, as conceived of in the 1950s, was imagined as a detachable object that materialised the object of the mother's desire. It circulated between mother and child in a dialectic that paved the way for the notion of the phallus as a signifier. The imaginary phallus is an object of a desire located beyond the child and with which the child tries to identify. The Oedipus complex entails renouncing the fantasy of becoming the imaginary phallus.

Finally, Lacan took the idea of the imaginary phallus further by developing the theoretical and technical implications of the idea of the phallus as a signifier, while revisiting the Freudian castration complex. For Freud, castration was not only the real "castration", but also the symbolic lack of an imaginary object. In short, castration could be understood as the relationship of desire with a primal *mark* comparable to a tattoo, to circumcision, or to signs branded on animals. This mark, the sign that sustains castration, later called S_1 by Lacan, can also be illustrated by examples of tattooing given in Freud's *Totem and Taboo* (1912–1913). In Lacan's later formulation, the phallus is no longer either a fantasy or an object, it becomes a signifier without a signified or the pure signifier of *jouissance* (Lacan [1960] 2006, 696).

Having explained terms and their logical operations, we need to ask: how can a hysteric, above all a hysterical woman, signify binary sexual difference with only *one* signifier, the phallus? This was the problem that complicated Dora's itinerary, her quest motivated by a desire to know about love and sex. In that sense, Dora was always asking a question about being: What is it to *be* a woman? Unable to answer or comprehend this, it was at a metaphoric level that her neurosis was to acquire its full meaning. Thus, Freud's failure with Dora was tied to his attempt to bring in a real *object*, a man whom she might love, that is Herr K., and not to work with her metaphors. As Lacan puts it: "Freud did not see that the introduction of Herr K. as a normalizing object of heterosexual love could only remain metaphorical, as a last attempt to comply with the law of symbolic exchanges" ([1956–1957] 1994, 146). Indeed, quite often the introduction of a real object, like the baby brother in the case of Margarethe, only impedes the possibility of displacement and substitution.

When Freud (1920) noticed Margarethe's violent "bitterness against men", he decided to break off the treatment and referred her to a female colleague for reasons he considered "obvious" (p. 164). Was it the case that Freud (1920) could not tolerate the young woman's repudiation of men? Perhaps it was his identification with her father, "an earnest, worthy man, at bottom very tender-hearted" (p. 149) that posed a problem. Freud nevertheless saw Margarethe's reawakened love for her father as positive transference. Was he suspicious because she brought him heterosexual "lying dreams" that tried both to please and to betray him (p. 166)? Freud concludes his description of Margarethe's pronounced "masculinity complex" with the declaration: "[s]he was in fact a feminist" (p. 166). It is quite striking that Freud qualifies Margarethe's repudiation of men and challenge of masculine authority as ideology. Some women, like the famous Anna O. (Bertha Pappenheim) reinvented themselves by feminism. Anna O.'s transformation from famous case study into women's rights activist is quite admirable. Yet, if Margarethe was trying to change the social condition of women, she was at a disadvantage, as Harris (1999) notes, "If 'she was in fact a feminist' she was a feminist quite without the support of feminism" (p. 157). The information one gathers in the biography confirms that if she was touched by feminism, she was not transformed. We see her always as a willing captive of her father's approval, with no indication of a desire to fight and challenge her own dependence, social status, or fears.

Was Freud reacting to his own family-romance conflict considering his daughter Anna's lesbian inclinations when dealing with Margarethe's same-sex love? Let us note that the Baroness Léonie Gessmann-Puttkamer, the "older" lady, was at the time 28 years old! Needless to say, it is obvious that Freud was full of contradictions; he both went along and broke with the prejudices of patriarchal thinking on femininity and homosexuality. A few paragraphs further, Freud offered this insight, still relevant today in current discussions of confusions between object choice and sexual identity:

> [t]he literature of homosexuality usually fails to distinguish clearly enough between questions of choice of object on the one hand, and of sexual characteristics and sexual attitude on the other, as though the answer to the former necessarily involved the answers to the latter.
>
> (1920, 170)

How to understand his abrupt interruption of the treatment? Its root may be Freud's initial scepticism about "treating" homosexuality, a scepticism that is reiterated at the end, when he stated that "it is not for psychoanalysis to solve the problem of homosexuality" (p. 171). Or was it that Freud could not continue this treatment of female homosexuality before he had solved the problem of femininity, this infamous "dark continent" that still eluded him?

Offered to Be Seen

When Lacan ([1962–1963] 2014) reopened Freud's "case of female homosexuality", it was in the context of the discussion of the function of the object that caused desire, which he designated with the letter *a* (pp. 122–123). This object emerged with brutal force in Margarethe's first suicide attempt, especially in view of the diverging version that has emerged in the Rieder and Voigt biography (2019, 13–14). Lacan interpreted Margarethe's defiance, strolling down the street in the arms of the lady, as an "acting out", which is when things are "offered to be seen" (*donné à voir*).

According to Freud, Margarethe's suicide attempt occurred shortly after she witnessed her father's anger, causing the lady to reject her. However, the biography offers a different perspective. In this version, Margarethe and the lady saw Margarethe's father accompanied by a colleague at a distance of about a block

away. Startled and panicked, Margarethe hastily fled down the street to avoid being noticed by her father. Upon her return a few minutes later, she found that her
father had already left, having boarded a trolley. This alternate account suggests
that Margarethe's father was unaware of her presence, while it was the lady who
observed the situation. Notably, the biography highlights the lady's criticism of
Margarethe, insinuating that her fear of her father's ire indicated insincerity. It was
this combination of the lady's reproach with the uncertainty around whether her
father had seen them or not which ultimately precipitated the suicide attempt. In
this version, the father's *blindness* played a pivotal role.

In reality, it is probable that the father did see his daughter as Thomas Gindele
(2003, 397) suggests, given that he was the one who brought her to the treatment,
and he likely provided Freud with his own account of the event. However, Margarethe's differing recollection adds emotional weight to her suicide attempt. While
Freud describes a disapproving look from her father as the catalyst for her actions,
Margarethe recalls seeing her father at the end of the street engaged in conversation
with a colleague before boarding a tramway. Fearful of being noticed, she fled from
the lady before realising her father's departure. Uncertain if he had seen her with
the baroness or chose to ignore her altogether, Margarethe's account introduces
ambiguity. Freud highlights an interesting aspect of the lady's rejection: her use of
language mirrored that of Margarethe's father and reiterated the same prohibition.

By throwing herself onto the tracks, Margarethe did three things at once: She
killed the imaginary gaze of the father that she had interiorised, she reinscribed a
symbolic father via her possible death (since the dead father is the symbolic father,
and this was the father with whom she identified), and she acted out in the real the
absolute seriousness of her affection for the lady. Thus, Margarethe's uncertainty
regarding whether her father had seen her end up disclosing an object, the gaze, in
all its importance. Symptomatically, the privileged position of the gaze as object
a reappeared in Freud's farewell to Margarethe at the end of treatment. He told
her: "You have such shrewd eyes. I would never want to have you as my enemy"
(Rieder and Voigt 2019, 55).

A Postfeminist Reading of Margarethe's Case

Margarethe's case history has been discussed at some length by Diana Fuss (1993,
1995, 1999) in an essay that has been often quoted and anthologised. Given Fuss's
reputation as a renowned deconstructive feminist, I find her critique exemplary.
Fuss (1995) is attentive to language and materiality, a tradition concerned with discerning the true meanings of "*gender* and *sexual difference*. Her point of departure
is an examination of "the cognitive paradigm of 'falling' which Freud provides in
this case study to 'explain' female homosexuality" (p. 57). Fuss contends that the
young woman's fall is not so much a fall as a regression, a "gravitational fall back
into a preoedipality" through a concomitant desire for the mother and identification
with the father. Fuss uses this as a springboard to investigate critically psychoanalytic theories that depict female homosexuality in terms of "pre-" something:

pre-oedipal, pre-symbolic, prelaw, premature, pre-sexual, and even pre-theoretical. All these tend to "position their subjects *as* foundational, primeval, primitive, and indeed as pre-subjects, before the normative, heterosexualising operations of the Oedipus complex" (p. 58; italics in the original). The problem that Fuss sees in Freud's approach therefore is bound up with the Oedipus complex in all its forms, not just with feminine sexuality.

Like Lacan, Fuss is sceptical of the way in which Freud explains the shift in Margarethe from a maternal attitude (wanting to *be* a mother) to a homosexual one (wanting to *have* a mother) as the result of her mother's late pregnancy and birth of a younger brother. Fuss questions the key role of the promise of a substitute object, challenging Freud's theory of femininity, a theory that is just sketched in this 1920 case and was expanded in the next decade with three crucial contributions.[4]

On this account, Fuss's project is quite worthwhile. Freud himself was aware of his theoretical shortcomings when elucidating the formation of sexual identity and, particularly, of feminine sexuality. Whereas an earlier stage of Freud's theoretical elaboration asserted that the Oedipus complex was similar for both sexes, his later texts on libidinal organisation stress differences in object choice, in the effects of the castration complex, and in the narcissistic investment of the genital organs. Freud's last works underline the fact that the first object for the girl is the mother, and that later variations will determine whether she can reach a feminine positioning via identifications that will guide object choice.

Thus, Fuss is unconvinced by Freud's explanation of the daughter's movement towards the mother, following what in 1920 was described by Freud as an "enigmatic disappointment" and in 1932 was theorised as an "inevitable disappointment". This generalisation was made in the 1932 lecture "Femininity", in which Freud put forward the idea of a "masculinity complex" in women as a regression from the attachment to the father.

Fuss (1995) questioned Freud's use of the word *regress* which she understood as a backward motion, as "a retrenchment rather than an advance, a retreat *from* the father rather than a move *toward* the mother" (p. 64; italics in the original). Fuss describes Freud's speculation about a displacement of the heterosexual daughter-father incest onto the mother as a disavowal of the homosexual daughter-mother incest (p. 64). She dismissed Freud's idea that for girls the "early masculinity complex" *is* the daughter-mother incest.

Against these strictures, one can adduce Lacan's idea that incest is always an incest with the mother, who stands for the first Other, the first *heteros*. The mother occupies the place of the sole incestuous object thanks to her primal role due to the state of helplessness in which the baby finds itself when born, a fact that makes it depend on an other (the mother) for its survival. But she is also from the Other sex, thus opening the way to the *heteros* of sex. The psychic importance of the mother can be shown by the devastating effects of maternal deficits for the child, as proven by the studies of René Spitz (1945, 1966) on hospitalism in which he studied institutionalised infants who failed to thrive physically and psychically despite adequate nutrition and health care. Similarly, Jenny Aubry (1983), a pioneer of child psychoanalysis in France, demonstrated that children who lacked adequate maternal care (often children who were separated from the mother or mother substitute and from their environment at birth) presented autistic characteristics and behaviours of self-aggression and self-mutilation. This chimes in with Lacan's analysis of the devastation caused by maternal deficits when the child is not the object of a particularised life desire, even if presented through the lack in the mother, it can neither develop nor get structured (Lacan [1969] 1990). The consequences of early maternal deficits can be catastrophic, but on the other hand, even if deficient, the separation from such important first love is not easy, especially for a girl. This sends us back to the question posed by Freud (1933) in his "Femininity" lecture: "How does a girl pass from her mother to an attachment to her father?" (p. 147).

The answer may address Fuss's criticism. The initial symmetry between boys and girls in their love for the mother ends when castration introduces a logic that distinguishes boys and girls in reference to a tertiary term, the phallus. The paternal prohibition works in a twofold manner: do not reintegrate your product (to the mother) and, you will not have sex with your mother (to the child). Under the dominance of phallic criteria, *boy* now means *having a penis* or *not without not having it*, *virile*, *being a man*, and so on. Similarly, the signifier *girl* acquires a phallic signification and loses its anatomical connotations to adopt other meanings, such as *feminine*, *mysterious*, *lacking*, *demure*, *beautiful*. For the boy, the phallus and castration resolve the Oedipal problems. For the girl, things are more complex. The resolution of the Oedipus complex orients both boys and girls towards a masculine position (both love the mother and have to renounce her).

Serge André (1999) assessed this early period of Freud's theorisation of femininity and contended that the girl, to avoid homosexuality and move to a male object, had to undergo "a change of sex" in fantasy (p. 173). To test the claim that homosexuality is inscribed in the structure of the feminine Oedipus complex and that a heterosexual object choice implied a change of sex in fantasy, André discussed the case of the young homosexual woman (pp. 173–184). Freud could never fully account for why not all girls go on to become homosexual. The so-called normal outcome of the Oedipus complex, the relation to the father, could be in fact re-editions of the earlier attachment to the mother.

Keeping One's Promise

Fuss rejects Freud's argument that the desire for the mother is a return to a "hated rival", a regression that would be caused by the frustration in her Oedipal inclinations for the father. She asks: "Why, in short, is the daughter's 'rivalry' assumed to be with the mother and not with the father?" (Fuss 1995, 62). According to Freud, in the resolution of the Oedipus complex, the girl resents her mother for having deprived her of a penis, and she will turn to her father in the hope that he will provide a child as a symbolic substitute for the penis. Fuss is absolutely right; Freud's theory of femininity ends in an impasse: The outcome of the feminine Oedipus is nothing other than a regression to the preoedipal connection to the mother.

Lacan's way out of this conundrum is first to question the efficacy of the Oedipus complex to understand femininity. It seems to explain so well boys' sexuality but does not seem to be fully operative in the case of girls. Lacan will put less emphasis on castration and to the claims it leads to, and more on the division that the primacy of the phallus creates for the girl. For Lacan, the privation of the phallus in the girl is the real lack of a symbolic object (the symbolic phallus); the missing penis is already a symbolic notion imposed onto the real, in which nothing is missing ([1956–1957] 1994, 210–211). Thus, the mother is deprived of an object that she actually never had. If there is anything perceived as lacking, what is absent is already the symbolic phallus, and the agent of privation is the imaginary father. As exemplified by Margarethe, the girl displaces onto her father the resentment she felt for her mother – for not giving her a penis – when he fails to provide the desired child.

According to Freud (1933, 1937), this resentment will be the moving force: it makes women desire a penis in sexual intercourse and want a child from a man. Lacan, however, claimed that no object can be sufficient because privation is imaginary: No matter how many children a woman may have, the dissatisfaction may persist because desire has no exact corresponding object. Then, the mother will desire other things beyond the children (like a lover, her job, watching a movie, and so on). The mother's dissatisfaction is propitious because it introduces the dialectics of desire that allow the child to see beyond the mother's desire. This helps the child look outside the dyad.

Let me emphasise this point: Fuss's anti-essentialist avoidance of the concept of the phallus gives the impression that she is not aware of the fact that children notice anatomical differences only after the symbolic event brought about by the threat of castration. Anatomy becomes then part of a mythical real that acquires signification on this second stage, when the values of the sex assigned at birth are structured and a sexual positioning is assumed. Finally, an object choice is made.

In Dora's case, the promise was that she could access the paternal phallus by way of Herr K., who stood out as an object of desire structured around his connection to Frau K. This is the promise that Herr K. broke in the scene by the lake. In this labyrinth of connections, when Herr K. made a clearer sexual advance, taking Dora in his arms while disavowing any interest in his wife, she slapped him in the face. He had said: "You know I get nothing out of my wife" (Freud 1905, 98). Lacan, following closely the syntax of the phrase in German ("*Ich habe nichts an meiner Frau*") noted that Herr K. was severing the previous circuit as if he had been telling Dora: "There is nothing in me of my wife." To add insult to injury, Dora may have heard the same complaint from her father's lips since we know that Dora's father used the exact phrase when he talked to Freud about Dora's mother (p. 26, fn. 106). Herr K.'s fateful confession suddenly short-circuited the circuit of desire sustained by the mediating function of the other woman. This is why when Freud first met Dora, she complained that her father had wronged her, and thus she required reparation; frustrated, torn by jealousy and resentment, she had moved to the level of demand.

Similarly, Freud (1920) claims that Margarethe's homosexuality was the result of a broken promise based on an exchange or economy of the gift. The lingering question is whether the *symbolic gift of a child* is equivalent to a woman's desire to have a child, and if that wish can be the same as her desire to become a mother. This is why Fuss (1995) is quite right to stress that Freud's case begins with the word *homosexuality* and concludes with the word *motherhood* (p, 66). Indeed, the missing word here would be *femininity*, a word that seems to remain out of reach not only for Freud but also for the unconscious.

The case of Margarethe can be understood in terms of frustration considered as a failure in the paternal discourse. For Freud, the love for the father was shaped by the default of a promise. In this case, the father's broken promise of a baby shattered Margarethe's trust in a symbolic chain of gift exchanges. Margarethe's tender, loving exaltation (*Schwärmerei*) of the fallen lady combined with her humble devotion reveal a dynamic of exchanges in which the young woman expected little and asked for nothing (Lacan [1956–1957] 1994, 101). Her lack of pretensions ("*che poco spera e nulla chiede*" ["hoping for little, wanting nothing"]) was rather a phobic "*noli me tangere*" ["do not touch me"] (Diamantis 2004, 60). The counterpoint to the strategy of demanding nothing from the baroness is that Margarethe was actually demanding something from the father. As with Dora, frustration made Margarethe move to the level of demand: She had been wronged and the father goes from being a symbolic father to an imaginary father. In her frustrated love, she identifies with the imaginary father who becomes the addressee of her demand for love, staged in the scene that he is forced to witness. As Freud (1920) puts it, Margarethe had been frustrated in "the wish to have a child by her father, for now she 'fell' through her father's fault" (p. 162). One may conclude that Margarethe did not simply *regress*, as Fuss claims, but rather that she *fell* into the barrenness of the real.

If, as she believed, the phallus was received by her mother (in German, *to receive* is *bekommen*), the same phallus had been denied to her, so that it fell (it falls, *es kommt nieder*). Nonetheless, her attempted suicide was at the same time – as the word itself reveals – a giving birth, that is, a symbolic parturition, an idea to which we will return. Freud noted that she was identified with the missing object: She became the baby she was denied. In her *niederkommen*, she was at once having the child and destroying herself, in a symbolic stillbirth. Whereas Dora remained in metaphoric substitution, Margarethe's desperate act was the last element in a long chain of displaced objects where actions speak louder than words.

Fuss, critical of Freud's study, denounces the limitations of the theory of female sexual inversion, a theory that she claims is based on a single case history. Yet, she falls into the same trap since she criticises Freud's theory of female sexuality from a single case history. She never proposes an alternative theory of female sexuality or of homosexuality. There is an element of truth in Jack Drescher's observation about the *pivotal role* that this 1920 Freud essay played in the psychoanalytic theory of female homosexuality and his reproach that "its biased views toward lesbians … became codified into the psychoanalytic canon" (Drescher 2001, 1447).

However, such so-called biases have issued from highly selective if not tendentious readings of Freud's theories of sexuality.

Fuss attacked Freud for reducing homosexuality to identification. As stated, her analysis of Freud's theory of female homosexuality is based on the paradigm of falling that she translates into the Latin *cadere* (to fall); this etymological connection then conjures up cadavers, an "insatiable oral drive", and a view of homosexuality as "identification in overdrive" (Fuss 1995, 77). Is this criticism itself in *overdrive*? Fuss's assessment of Freud's theory of homosexuality focuses on the verb *niederkommen* ("to fall", or to be delivered of a child), a verb that had been given to Freud by Margarethe. Freud did not employ it to *explain* female homosexuality, as Fuss argues, but to analyse the logic of her suicidal attempt. Here, Fuss's reading strays from the close textual attention that her critique would require. As a result, she gives the impression of not knowing Freud very well or of wilfully distorting the letter of his texts. How else can one make sense of her claim that

> for Freud every fall into homosexuality is *inherently suicidal* since the 'retreat' from preoedipality entails not only the loss of desire but the loss of a fundamental relation to the world into which desire permits entry – the world of sociality, sexuality, and subjectivity.
>
> (p. 77; italics in the original)

Fuss criticises Freud for not having elaborated a theory of homosexual desire. She dismisses the fact that Freud did not use desire as a theoretical concept (as Lacan did) and that, properly speaking, Freud did not have a theory of desire, homo or hetero. In a series of curious interpretive inversions, Fuss aligns object choice with heterosexuality and identification with homosexuality, believing that for Freud "desire is the province and privilege of heterosexuals, homosexuals are portrayed as hysterical identifiers and expert mimics" (Fuss 1999, 71). Rather than follow Freud's development of his theory of identification from the Oedipus complex to "Totem and Taboo" (Freud 1912–1913) and "Moses and Monotheism" (Freud 1939), Fuss treats it as a consistent whole and then attacks its coherence: "Freud in spectacular circular fashion, resubmits homosexuality to its own alleged entropic 'tendencies,' so that 'homo' subsumes 'sexuality' and identification incorporates desire" (Fuss 1999, 71–72). On the other hand, Fuss is right to refuse the idea that homosexuality would appear as a regression when the choice of maternity is frustrated. Indeed, she poses the question of whether this might be a case of identity formation, of homosexuality versus motherhood, or of same-sex desire and same-sex identification. Fuss's essay convincingly exposes the limitations of Freud's Oedipus model, showing how identity and desire may not always overlap.

If Freud can be blamed for not having elaborated a theory of homosexual desire beyond his contention of regression to a primeval identification, Fuss's essay does not escape similar charges. Since she did not propose an alternative theory of homosexuality, her claims become increasingly contradictory. In a sweeping gesture, she asserted that female homosexuality is psychoanalysis' very foundation, contending that out of Freud's six completed case studies, two are studies of object choice inversion in women (Fuss 1999, 59). Fuss neglected the fact that Freud treated more than six patients during his whole analytic career. Besides the four pre-psychoanalytic cases published in the *Studies on Hysteria*, none of them on homosexuality, there is evidence (reports or autobiographies, letters, and interviews of analysands, letters by Freud, published works by Freud, and clinical records of subsequent treatment) that Freud treated *at least* 43 patients between 1907 and 1939 (Lynn and Vaillant 1998). Similarly Fuss claimed that Lacan's early focus on paranoia was because "Lacan was interested only in *homosexual women*" (1999, 56, italics in the original). Lacan's interest was not in homosexual women but in paranoia. While one may indeed argue whether the Papin sisters' incest that led to a notorious massacre should be considered as *homosexual* (Christine Papin believed that in a former life she was her sister's husband), at least in the case of Aimée, the paranoiac patient studied by Lacan in his early-career dissertation, her infatuation with an actress was clearly not homosexual but self-punishing (Roudinesco, 1997).

Like Judith Butler, Fuss (1999) thinks that in Freud's model, the child's homosexual desire for the parent of the same sex is a fundamental, yet disposable component of desire, a component that has to be repudiated and repressed. According to her, the "inessentiality" of homosexuality reflects a secondary reaction formation against the attraction of psychoanalysis to an economy of the same (homo) and a fascination with its own origins. Yet, if one pushes the thesis to its rigorous conclusion, it becomes absurd as it implies that from the start girls only love their mothers and boys only their fathers, and that they repress that homosexual first choice to become heterosexual. This repressed homosexual primer would reduce all sexual forms to heterosexual choices; that is, if two people of the same sex desire one another, one has to have identified with the opposite sex, thus reproducing a heterosexual matrix within homosexual desire.

While one cannot seriously say that Freud ever dehumanised homosexuals, one can grant that Freud lacks a full theory of feminine homosexuality, a theoretical failing that led to a well-known controversy on femininity. For a long time, Freud answered the question, "*Was will das Weib?*" ("What does a woman want") (Jones 1955, 421) by saying that he knew well what women wanted. He called that desire "penis envy": since they did not *have* it, they chose the man who *had* it. But, in 1923, Freud took a dramatic turn and admitted that he had been wrong (Freud 1923b). It is not a penis but love for the mother that the girl wants, and for that, like the boy, she has to renounce something in the Oedipal struggle. Is the female homosexual, for Freud, a girl with an arrested psychosexual development as Fuss (1999) claims? The details of Freud's reversal and the understanding of regression from object choice to identification have stirred a long debate in feminist criticism. The debate has not been closed and keeps eliciting more conflicting views.

Tiresias Knew

In an influential essay dating from 1980, Adrienne Rich turned the argument of heterosexual object choice on its head: If the first erotic bond is to the mother, she asked, could not the "natural" sexual orientation of both men and women be toward women (1986, 23–75)? In fact, there is nothing *natural* about either heterosexuality or homosexuality. More recently, commenting on the "heterosexual matrix" that prevails in our society, Judith Butler (1997) discussed the predicaments of a culture that struggles to mourn the loss of the homosexual –attachment (pp. 132–150). Butler then stated that any sexual position is acquired, at least partially, not through mourning but rather as a repudiation of homosexual attachments. Concerning femininity, she asserted that "the girl becomes a girl through being subject to a prohibition which bars the mother as an object of desire and installs that barred object as a part of the ego, indeed, as a melancholic identification" (p. 136).

Fundamentally, Butler has challenged the idea that sexual identity is built around object choice. She wrote: "If one is a girl to the extent that one does not want a girl, then wanting a girl will bring being a girl into question", adding that within this matrix, homosexual desire challenges gender (p. 136). Lacan ([1958c] 2006) acknowledged the inability of psychoanalysts, male and female alike, to elucidate feminine sexuality with a challenge: "A convention on female sexuality is not about to cause to weight upon us the threat of Tiresias fate" (p. 613). In 1972–1973, Lacan argued that castration could not fully account for the feminine positioning because femininity was a position regarding sex not fully determined by the phallus ([1972–1973] 1999, 72). There was nothing mysterious about feminine sexuality; mystery was a fantasy to cloud over the lack of a rapport between the sexes. The problem of femininity is, for Lacan, centred around how the phallic function (which works in an asymmetric manner for each gendered sexual positioning) is unconsciously signified and depends on how each subject acknowledges their subjection to the law of sexual difference.

Let us return to the scene that precipitated the suicide attempt of Margarethe. The young woman was, as Judith Butler would say, "performing her gender", parading her *knight* persona in a scene carefully staged for her father's gaze. When the lady discovers in the street that the whole scene was a spectacle of passionate devotion with the purpose of infuriating the father, she brutally rejects Margarethe. The lady refuses to continue the relationship with the young woman not just because she sees a public display of romantic courtship addressed to the father as a rebellious transgression, but also because, echoing the young woman's father, she recognises her behaviour as tarnishing her own reputation (Freud 1920, 125). Above all, it was because she suddenly became aware of her secondary role in a scene performed mostly for Margarethe's father, that the baroness found her part unacceptable. Like a spurned prima donna, she left the scene. Here, there was no more room for laughter as the parody has rung too true.

The performance enacted by Margarethe had posited the baroness as a capricious master not bound by moral laws. For her, the baroness was the mythical *She,* the Woman, whose legendary primordial repression constitutes the symbolic order. Margarethe was promoting the Woman to the level of the Name-of-the-Father to make up for her father's deficiency. She performed a scene in which she could find in her lady an absolute phallus with which she could signify her sexuality. This calls up the idea of Woman as a Name-of-the-Father in a logic of supplementarity that organises *jouissance* according to the tangled knots of a *sinthome*. For the moment, I would like to stay with Lacan's double notion of acting out – a subject's performance of a scene for the gaze of the Other – and *passage à l'acte* (passage to the act, a sudden impulsive act). These two terms, which I will explain below, also address the premises that provide the foundation for Butler's ideas of gender as performative. Since both Dora and Margarethe present cases of women's *virile* inclinations (*männliches Typus*) whose sexual object is someone of the same sex, they offer a good ground to test Butler's ideas of sex and gender. This allows us to reframe the critiques of the work of Lacan and Freud by queer and feminist theory.

In Love, Gender Is Irrelevant

We have seen that Fuss's model of gravitational pushes and pulls made the mistake of collapsing object choice and sexual identity. To avoid this slippage, one needs to reopen the case of Margarethe by taking into account her *significant other*. As Lacan noted in a seminar in which homosexuality was a key issue to understand feminine sexuality, as far as love is concerned, gender seems irrelevant. He said: "*Quand on aime il ne s'agit pas de sexe*" ["When one loves, it has nothing to do with gender"] (Lacan [1972–1973] 1999, 25). With this in mind, I follow the grid proposed by Lacan ([1962–1963] 2014) in a passage of the seminar on *Anxiety* in which he calls the suicidal attempt a "passage to the act" and also describes Margarethe's infatuation with the lady as an acting out.

The pair *acting out* and *passage to the act* can serve to analyse the scene of Margarethe's suicide as a performance staging an encounter with the object cause of desire (object *a*), suddenly emerging unfiltered by desire and deprived of the veil of the fantasy. Margarethe's suicidal attempt was a ploy that attempted, at least temporarily, to ward off anxiety. Although anxiety is at work in both the acting out and the passage to the act, Lacan establishes a clear distinction between them. While both are strategies deployed against anxiety, in the acting out the subject remains in the scene, whereas in the passage to the act the subject leaves the scene altogether. Margarethe's acting out was addressed to the Other, first taken as the father. The passage to the act, however, implies a flight from the Other into the dimension of the real; it is an exit from the symbolic network, bringing along a dissolution of the social bond. It is a message addressed to anyone and no one in particular and entails a disintegration of the subject, who for a moment is turned into a pure object *a*, a leftover of signification, and falls from the scene (Lacan [1962–1963] 2014, 114–130).

The acting out of Margarethe occurred before she began the treatment, and it functioned as the event that precipitated being brought to analysis. This evokes Lacan's claim that the acting out was "transference without analysis" (p. 125) that is, a "wild transference" (p. 126). Unlike certain symptoms that may not beg for an interpretation because they are not a call to the Other but pure *jouissance* addressed to no one, an acting out always calls for an interpretation (p. 147). Roberto Harari writes that acting out is untamed transference insofar as it questions and over-whelms the subject to a much greater extent than the symptom: "In acting out, we must take into account that the subject is experiencing phallic jouissance" (2001, 85). In that sense, an acting out has a stronger power of demand than the symptom: "It is a peremptory demand for interpretation, given the shattering it bears" (p. 85). Whether gender is a performance, an acting out, or a *passage à l'acte*, what matters for a psychoanalyst is the negotiation between the subject and the object *a* with which the performance plays. Following Butler's (1990, 1997) theoretical progression, we will find in mourning a good example of the complex circuit of the object as it determines subjective positions.

Gender and Melancholy

Butler (1997) builds gender on a certain conception of melancholy that derives from Freud's "Mourning and Melancholia". As is well known, Freud differenti-ates melancholy from mourning: Mourning refers to an experience of grieving or of working through an external identifiable loss (a loved person, an ideal), while melancholy corresponds to a state of endless grief that develops into a morbid condition (the ego identifies with the lost object itself). Freud contends that the mourner gives up the lost object by "offering the ego the inducement of continu-ing to live" (Freud 1917, 257). Grief work (*Trauerarbeit*) is a task that allows a certain economy to be restored; one attachment is severed to make others possible. Butler's model, however, describes a subject unable to forget or repress, incapable of grieving the loss of the homosexual object, ill-equipped to cut ties and move on.

Let us distinguish more clearly Butler's (1997) position from that of Fuss (1993, 1995, 1999). Fuss attacked the Freud (1917) of "Mourning and Melancholia" and his claim that the loss of an object produces a regression to identification which she argued neglected the revised theory of mourning offered six years after "Mourning and Melancholia" in "The Ego and the Id". In "The Ego and the Id", Freud suggests that mourning is not always possible: with very significant objects, the process of mourning may never be completed (Freud 1923a, 31). Freud's theoretical turn can be traced back to his daughter Sophie's death. In a 1929 letter to Binswanger, Freud mentioned the persistence of mourning and generalised the experience of having lost his daughter nine years earlier:

> We know that the acute sorrow we feel after such a loss will run its course, but also that we will remain inconsolable, and will never find a substitute. No mat-ter what may come to take its place, even should it fill that place completely, it yet remains something else. And that is how it should be. It is the only way of perpetuating a love that we do not want to abandon.
>
> (Freud 1929, 196)

If the people we love deeply are eminently irreplaceable, the possibility of true mourning seems challenged. In 1923, Freud redefines the ego's character as "a precipitate of abandoned object-cathexes", that is, an embodied history of lost erotic attachments (1923a, 29). This is the claim that Butler follows when she contends that no final severance of attachments "could take place without dissolving the ego" (1997, 196).

Butler is much closer to the Freud of "The Ego and the Id" who often contradicted the claims in "Mourning and Melancholia". While Fuss criticises Freud's use of regression, for Butler, it is regression that allows women to come closer to the nexus of attachment lost in the compulsory production of heterosexuality. For Butler, the inability to accept the loss of the homosexual attachment comes in the way of the possibility of a regression and stalls a progression to the next object; as a consequence, subjects remain trapped in a primeval melancholy.

Identification with the Rival

In "The Ego and the Id", Freud surprises the reader by stating that it is not bisexuality but identification with the rival object that governs the formation of "normal" sexual identity (thus contradicting Fuss's assumptions once more). In his discussion of the "simple positive Oedipus complex in a boy", which is characterised by an "ambivalent attitude to his father and an object-relation of a solely affectionate kind to his mother" (Freud 1923a, 32), Freud argues that to cope with the loss of the mother, the boy substitutes this maternal object cathexis regressing to two forms of identification: "either an identification with his mother or an intensification of his identification with his father" (p. 32). In his theorising, Freud questions his own proposition: he suggests the "more normal" identifications emerging in the Oedipus complex "are not what we should have expected since they do not introduce the abandoned object into the ego" (p. 32). In the case of "the more complete Oedipus complex, which is twofold, positive and negative" and due to "the bisexuality originally present in children" (p. 33), the boy may not simply be ambivalent about his father and affectionate with his mother; he may behave like a girl facing his father and be jealous and hostile with his mother. Freud, however, continues to imply that identification with the rival constitutes the norm. Identification preserves the loved and hated rival within the ego, but an ego subject to the violently critical, obscene, and ferocious superego.

If we return to Margarethe, we can see that she appeared to have substituted her love choice for her Oedipal rival. Indeed, Freud claimed that "analysis revealed beyond all shadow of doubt that the lady-love was a substitute for—her mother" (1920, 156). It is true that the lady was not herself a mother, yet Freud asserts that for Margarethe "[m]otherhood [w]as a *sine qua non* in her love object" (p. 156), even when her own mother favoured her sons and was not very kind to her. Freud suggests that when the girl was experiencing a revival of the Oedipus complex, she suffered a great disappointment. She had already developed a strong affection for a little boy whom she would often see in a playground. She was conscious of her wish to have a baby boy when her mother gave birth to her youngest brother. Her true disappointment came from the fact that, being unable to become the mother of her father's child, she repudiated her wish for a child and threw the baby out with the bath water, as it were, and rejected femininity altogether. The flaw in her logic was the following: being a mother was the only answer to the question, "what is to be a woman?" Since she was unable to be a mother, she could not be a woman. Then, according to Freud, a major transformation occurred – Margarethe became a man. She "changed into a man and took her mother in place of her father as the object of her love" (p. 158). As her relation to her mother was hostile, she was able to overcompensate via a substitute mother to whom she could be passionately attached.

The Rieder and Voigt biography describes Gretl's mother as distant and uninterested, "lenient to the point of indifference" (2019, 11). She discovered that by letting her mother know about her homosexual inclinations, she would leave men to her mother; thus she would overcome the mother-daughter rivalry by avoiding any antagonism, or as Freud said, she decided to "retire in favour of her mother" (Freud 1920, 158).

Her father's dislike of her homosexuality reinforced the success of the strategy – Margarethe could both regain her mother's love and take revenge on her father. She wanted the father to know because her behaviour followed a retaliatory principle. In effect, according to Freud, she thought: "Since you have betrayed me, you must put up with my betraying you" (p. 159). The broken promise, however, got re-enacted in the transference. Unhappily, Freud missed the opportunity of an analytic intervention that would have allowed the young woman to abandon a purely egoic discourse and engage with her unconscious desire. This moment is described as one of "positive transference" (p. 164) and relates to a period in the treatment at which Margarethe had a series of dreams of getting cured, longing for husband and children. Freud did not believe these dreams, declaring them "false or hypocritical". He concluded that Margarethe "intended to deceive me as she habitually deceived her father" (p. 165).

This fits with Freud's general description of Margarethe. Freud had painted her as someone who was "full of deceitfulness", who "disdained no means of deception, no excuses, and no lies" to get what she wanted (1920, 148). While he was quite suspicious of her, the deceiving dreams first had positive elements; he evokes these with a dose of scepticism:

> Beside the intention to mislead me, the dreams partly expressed the wish to win my favour; they were also an attempt to gain my interest and my good opinion— perhaps in order to disappoint me all the more thoroughly later on.
>
> (p. 165)

Gretl's lying dreams had a purpose, not only to deceive him just as she deceived her father, but also to make a promise to Freud that she knew she was going to break. This is how she would re-enact her own drama of frustration in the transference.

No doubt Freud felt wronged and imaginarily wounded. He reacted strongly to the lies which he saw as a provocation that precipitated the termination of the treatment. What Freud missed in this situation is that the unconscious usually lies to tell a truth. Margarethe's unconscious had lied to expose the truth of the promise that the father could not fulfil. The main issue in this case was not the object (whether a baby, a husband, or a cure) as much as the promise. Freud's decoding of this message would have allowed for the constitution of a demand of analysis in what up to then was just a preliminary stage. Indeed, Freud exposed the deception, but he missed its symbolic value as a message; therefore, he fell as well into the trap, he "fell through her father's fault" (p. 162). If Margarethe was staging an acting out for Freud, she was providing her analyst with a unique belvedere onto her *object cause of desire* because, as we have seen, the acting out as such is a scene that makes the *objet a* appear. Freud was not aware that in his position as analyst he was actually playing the role of object cause of desire. He simply fulfilled the destiny of the *objet a*, which is to fall: "The *a*, the object, falls. That fall is primal. The diversity of forms taken by that object of the fall ought to be related to the manner in which the desire of the Other is apprehended by the subject" (Lacan [1963] 1999, 85).

For Lacan, there is no doubt: Here, Freud makes a mistake, he "errs when he regards himself as the object aimed at in reality by the negative transference" (Lacan [1958a] 2006, 534). The broken promise was related to an object supposed to guarantee the movement from the mother to the father. Her intention was not to betray her father but to denounce the deception that Margarethe had experienced. Freud had missed a chance to truly start the analysis when he ended it. "What a pity it had to be broken off!" was the conclusion of Lou Andreas-Salomé after reading the case (Pfeiffer 1972, 102). She told Freud: "Behind the negative transference to you there lay hidden no doubt the original positive transference to the father. Would not this original basis come to light eventually in the acting out of the negative transference?" (p. 102). Her critique went to the heart of the matter: Freud blamed everything on negative transference, making the superficial assumption that it was all a "virile protest". This gesture was in fact more Adlerian than Freudian. Andreas-Salomé was openly sceptical about the hypothesis that the young woman became homosexual and was ready to commit suicide to take revenge on the father. This is, however, how Ernest Jones read the case, arguing that her homosexuality was to take revenge on her father, and that the suicide attempt was motivated by an identification with the father as the lost object (Jones 1955, 279).

Margarethe's negative transference was constituted by her hate for masculinity which was necessary to assume her sexual identity. If Freud had been able to tolerate the moment of negative transference and, instead of breaking off the treatment had taken the broken promise as a signifier of the Other, he could have turned the tables in the transference. Then, by working around the unkept promise implied by the "lying" dreams, he could have engaged the young woman in her desire, thus transforming an imaginary wound into a necessary lack. If, as Lacan ([1962–1963] 2014, 128–129) argues, Margarethe was telling the truth from the veiled position of a lie, she was already then negotiating castration by talking from a position of semblance, of make-believe.

Let us take a last look at Freud's theory that at the end of the latency phase the promise of a penis substitute is expected from a man who will always disappoint the girl, never fulfilling its promise. This is because he is no other than the father, whose exclusion is always demanded by the laws of exogamy. Taking a Freudian-Lacanian look at the logic of female homosexuality, Gérard Pommier (2000) offers a genealogy that slightly differs from Freud's but that applies handsomely to Margarethe's case. Pommier links female homosexuality with castration anxiety and its denial. His reconstructed logic goes as follows: The father refuses to give the penis to his daughter and has to physically reject her; otherwise, he would commit incest and cease being a father. This rejection may be greeted by violence and rebellion, which is often seen in the period preceding female homosexuality. Only love will be able to appease the castration anxiety thus unleashed and replace penis envy. Hence, the daughter will love a woman like a man, and she will acquire a penis vicariously. Female homosexual love, according to Pommier, would stem from a fantasy of masculinisation. Sexuality would then turn phallic by focusing on the clitoris.

For all its clarity, Pommier's (2000) systematisation does not fully explain Margarethe's sexuality who comes across as someone who has rejected sexuality altogether – she rejects her own femininity and repudiates masculinity while playing the part of the devoted knight toward her baroness. In her biography, a photograph shows her in male period costume that makes her look like an eighteenth-century *roué*, which seems to indicate that, for her, femininity was a transgressive virile disguise. Indeed, Margarethe had a hard time becoming a woman. Freud confirmed that she had rejected the sexual advances of a lesbian of her age and generally "had a physical repulsion to the idea of any sexual intercourse" (Freud 1920, 153). According to the biography, during her life, Margarethe experienced profound aversion to intimate sexual contact with male and female lovers alike (Rieder and Voigt 2019). Margarethe's disgust towards sex reminds us of classical hysteria. The young woman assumed in her behaviour towards her love object "the masculine part" (Freud 1920, 154) and "could not conceive of any other way of being in love" (p. 153) with a mother. Was the young woman wondering, "What is a woman?" or more pointedly, "What am I for my mother?"

The Child of an Acquaintance

It is in this context that Marcianne Blévis (2004) paid attention to the excessive love that Margarethe's mother, Emma, had for her sons and the detestation that she flaunted towards her daughter, an attitude that she kept even on her deathbed. "I think my mother is so beautiful, and I do everything for her, but she only loves my brothers" Margarethe recalls telling Freud (Rieder and Voigt 2019, 40). Blévis describes it as the delirious jealousy of Margarethe's mother, a jealousy that determined and constituted the homosexuality linking mother and daughter.

Indeed, the biography documents many painful instances of rejection. On one particularly humiliating occasion, which happened the year before the treatment with Freud, Margarethe and her mother were staying at a health spa, a place that Emma Csillag visited frequently to cure her nervous problems such as anxieties and fears. Away from her husband, Emma seemed much happier, enjoying the attention she commanded and behaving, to Margarethe's embarrassment, as if she were not a married woman. One of her admirers, struck by Gretl's beauty, congratulated the mother on having such a beautiful daughter. She responded to the compliment by claiming that Margarethe was not her daughter but "the child of an acquaintance" (Rieder and Voigt 2019, 42). Sobbing, Margarethe ran and locked herself in her room and spent the following days alone and inconsolable, refusing to speak to her mother (p. 42). The daughter understood the message.

In view of this interaction, which took place before the suicidal attempt that brought her to treatment, Gretl's predicament can be understood in terms of trying to give birth not to the Oedipal father's child, as Freud claims, but to herself. Margarethe was not suffering from a frustrated desire to receive a child from her father but rather was positioned outside the lineage, excluded by her mother. By claiming that Margarethe was not her daughter, the mother exiles her daughter from the family system of kinship.

The mother's wish to appear as the only desirable beauty also led to a deterioration of Margarethe's sexuality. Margarethe's symptoms can be interpreted as an attempt to repress maternal *jouissance* in the hope of salvaging her subjective and sexual identity from the mother's jealousy as well as a manifestation that despite "being of good birth as she was", (Freud 1920, 153), she was not properly born. Her suicide was a traumatic, aborted attempt at birthing herself.

When Freud tried to justify his having interrupted the treatment, he adduced the fact that he had become aware that Margarethe "transferred to [him] the sweeping repudiation of men which had dominated her ever since the disappointment she has suffered from her father" (p. 164). This is the repudiation of masculinity that has triggered the interest of feminists and queer theorists. Lacan maintains that observation shows that female homosexuality "is oriented by a disappointment that strengthens the axis of the demand for love" ([1958b] 2006, 583). Over and over again, Freud insisted that for the girl the threat of castration is experienced as a fear of loss of love.

Freud neglected the importance of love for Margarethe, a love that is directed to something beyond the phallus. Margarethe wanted to find in her father's gaze the love that would compensate for the privation of the phallus. As we have seen, not only did her father betray her, but she had to withdraw and let her mother enjoy men exclusively. And to complicate matters, her mother disowns her, declaring that Margarethe is not her daughter but the child of an acquaintance, making her an outsider to the family history. Did her mother appear positioned as the exception, as the woman who enjoys all the men? That would mean that Margarethe's mother was in the place of an x that did not fall under the law of castration. Did Margarethe reject her femininity as a way of refusing her mother as an exception? This assertion would imply that there exists at least one x that is not submitted to the phallic function; it is the exception that sustains the universal that is the male norm that entails for all men to be submitted to the phallic function by way of castration. Did Margarethe sacrifice her so-called normal femininity by choosing an angelic femininity? Indeed, her serene avoidance of the pleasures of the flesh calls up the figure of the angel, that is, an identity not based on sex. The angel is an asexual creature, outside time, and hence immortal. As a messenger, the angel invokes the annunciation of something. Lacan suggested that this figure helps us visualise the gap between the symbolic and the real, between the boundary of the sexual symbolic body and the real of the flesh ([1972–1973] 1999, 8–9). Angels are supposed to be in a state of perpetual bliss, a bliss that leaves nothing to be desired. Angels do not desire; they render a service – they love. Thus, we can say that Margarethe made a semblance of homosexuality, serially worshipping the women she loved, thereby negotiating her castration and reducing love to its declaration. Her suicidal gestures appear as the desperate attempts of someone not fully born to birth herself. Here, I consider death as a destructive force that paradoxically allows for a re-birth. Clinical work opens a path towards figuring out how to live with the death drive which paradoxically renders life possible. Here, death emerges not as the opposite of life but rather as a condition for life.

Acknowledgements

This chapter revisits my discussion of the case in *Please Select Your Gender: From the Invention of Hysteria to the Democratizing of Transgenderism* (Gherovici 2010, 93–129).

Notes

1 This case is Freud's (1920) case, "The Psychogenesis of a Case of Homosexuality in a Woman". Despite its clumsy title the syntax and style of which suggest a dry medical report, it was considered by Lacan ([1956–1957] 1994) as "one of the most brilliant texts of Freud", although he immediately added that it was "also one of the most disquieting cases", that it even seemed "archaic" or "out of fashion" (p. 94).
2 Much information on this fascinating treatment has been made available through the publication in German, with translations into French, Spanish, and English of a narrative biography of the protagonist of this case. Giving her the pseudonym Sidonie Csillag, Ines Rieder and Diana Voigt (2019) chronicle the life of Freud's patient who died in 1999 at the age of 99. After her death, her real name was disclosed as Margarethe Trautenegg, née Csonka. *Csillag* in Hungarian means "star" while *Csonka* translates as "mutilated". In October 2004, the research material used by Rieder and Voigt to construct the biography of "Sidonie Csillag" (a large photo collection, personal documents, and numerous interviews with Margarethe Csonka) was donated to the Sigmund Freud Museum in Vienna by the authors of the biography.
3 Harriet Mossop (in the lecture "Moving towards *Heartstopper* melancholy: Queer phenomenological and erotohistoriographic readings of the lives of four women from the history of psychoanalysis", unpublished paper) notes that there has been a scarcity of stories of queer and trans people in psychoanalysis. Sidonie's case is gradually getting some overdue attention. See *Sigmund Freud and his Patient Margarethe Csonka: A Case of Homosexuality in a Woman in Modern Vienna* (Shapira 2023).

4 The crucial texts in which Freud expounds his theory of femininity are "Some Psychical Consequences of the Anatomical Distinction Between the Sexes" (Freud 1925), "Female Sexuality" (Freud 1931), and "Femininity" (Freud 1933).

References

Aflalo-Lebovits, Agnès. (1984). "Sur le cas de la jeune homosexuelle". *Analytica Revue*, 3,: 23–42.

André, Serge. (1999). *What Does a Woman Want?* New York: Other Press.

Aubry, Jenny. (1983). *Enfance abandonnée*. Paris: Métailié.

Blévis, Marcianne. (2004). "La mère de la 'jeune homosexuelle' mise à nu par ses célibataires même". *Les Lettres de la S.P.F.*, 12, 93–107.

Butler, Judith. (1990). *Gender Trouble: Feminism and the Subversion of Identity*. New York: Routledge.

Butler, Judith. (1997). "Melancholy Gender/Refused Identification". In *The Psychic Life of Power: Theories in Subjection*, pp. 132–150. Stanford, CA: Stanford University Press.

Diamantis, I. (2004). "La prudence de la chair: Homosexualité et phobie". *Les Lettres de la S.P.F.*, 12, 51–64.

Drescher, Jack. (2001). "That Obscure Subject of Desire: Freud's Female Homosexual Revisited: Review". *Journal of the American Psychoanalytic Association*, 49, 1447–1450.

Freud, Sigmund. (1905). "Fragment of an Analysis of a Case of Hysteria". In *The Standard Edition of the Complete Psychological Works of Sigmund Freud*, translated by James Strachey, vol. 7, pp. 1–122. London: Hogarth, 1955.

Freud, Sigmund. (1912–1913). "Totem and Taboo". In *The Standard Edition of the Complete Psychological Works of Sigmund Freud*, translated by James Strachey, vol. 13, pp. 1–164. London: Hogarth, 1955.

Freud, Sigmund. (1917). "Mourning and Melancholia". In *The Standard Edition of the Complete Psychological Works of Sigmund Freud*, translated by James Strachey, vol. 14, pp. 237–258. London: Hogarth, 1955.

Freud, Sigmund. (1920). "Psychogenesis of a Case of Homosexuality in a Woman". In *The Standard Edition of the Complete Psychological Works of Sigmund Freud*, translated by James Strachey, vol. 18, pp. 145–172. London: Hogarth, 1955.

Freud, Sigmund. (1923a). "The Ego and the Id". In *The Standard Edition of the Complete Psychological Works of Sigmund Freud*, translated by James Strachey, vol. 19, pp. 1–66, London: Hogarth, 1955.

Freud, Sigmund. (1923b). "The Infantile Genital Organisation". In *The Standard Edition of the Complete Psychological Works of Sigmund Freud*, translated by James Strachey, vol. 19, pp. 141–145, London: Hogarth, 1955.

Freud, Sigmund.(1925). "Some Psychical Consequences of the Anatomical Distinction between the Sexes". In *The Standard Edition of the Complete Psychological Works of Sigmund Freud*, translated by James Strachey, vol. 19, pp. 248–258. London: Hogarth, 1955.

Freud, Sigmund. (1929). Letter from Freud to Ludwig Binswanger, April 11, 1929. In *The Sigmund Freud-Ludwig Binswanger Correspondence, 1908–1938*, 50: 196.

Freud, Sigmund. (1931). "Female Sexuality". In *The Standard Edition of the Complete Psychological Works of Sigmund Freud*, translated by James Strachey, vol. 21, pp. 221–244, London: Hogarth, 1955.

Freud, Sigmund. (1933). "Femininity". In *New Introductory Lectures on Psychoanalysis*. In *The Standard Edition of the Complete Psychological Works of Sigmund Freud*, translated by James Strachey, vol. 22, pp. 112–135, London: Hogarth, 1955.

Freud, Sigmund. (1937). "Analysis Terminable and Interminable". In *The Standard Edition of the Complete Psychological Works of Sigmund Freud*, translated by James Strachey, vol. 23, pp. 209–254, London: Hogarth, 1955.

Freud, Sigmund. (1939). "Moses and Monotheism". In *The Standard Edition of the Complete Psychological Works of Sigmund Freud*, translated by James Strachey, vol. 23, pp. 1–140, London: Hogarth, 1955.

Freud, Sigmund and Weiss, Eduardo. (1975). *Lettres sur la pratique analytique*. Paris: Privat.

Fuss, Diana. (1993). "Fallen Women: Identification, Desire, and 'A Case of Homosexuality in a Woman'". In M. Warner (ed.), *Fear of a Queer Planet: Queer Politics and Social Theory*, pp. 42–68. Minneapolis, MN: University of Minnesota Press.

Fuss, Diana.(1995). "Fallen Women: 'The Psychogenesis of a Case of Homosexuality in a Woman'". In *Identification Papers: Readings on Psychoanalysis, Sexuality, and Culture*, pp. 57–82. New York: Routledge.

Fuss, Diana. (1999). "Fallen Women: "The Psychogenesis of a Case of Homosexuality in a Woman". In R. Lesser and E. Schoenberg (eds), *That Obscure Subject of Desire: Freud's Female Homosexual Revisited*, pp. 54–75. New York: Routledge.

Gherovici, Patricia (2010), *Please Select Your Gender: From the Invention of Hysteria to the Democratizing of Transgenderism*. New York: Routledge.

Gindele, Thomas. (2003b). Postface: Freud, Lacan, Sidonie. In I. Rieder and D. Voigt (eds), *Sidonie Csillag: Homosexuelle chez Freud, lesbienne dans le siècle*, pp. 395–400. Paris: Epel.

Harari, Roberto. (2001). *Lacan's Seminar on Anxiety: An Introduction*. New York: Other Press.

Harris, Adrienne. (1999). "Gender as Contradiction". In *That Obscure Object of Desire: Freud's Female Homosexual Revisited*, edited by R. Lesser and E. Schoenberg, pp. 156–179. London: Routledge.

Jones, Ernest. (1955). *The Life and Work of Sigmund Freud*, vol. II: *1901–1919: Years of Maturity*. New York: Basic Books.

Lacan, Jacques. (1955–1956). *The Psychoses*. In *The Seminar of Jacques Lacan, Book III*, translated by Russell Grigg, edited by Jacques-Alain Miller. London: W.W. Norton & Co, 1993.

Lacan, Jacques. (1956–1957). *La relation d'objet*. In *Le séminaire de Jacques Lacan, Livre IV*. Paris: Editions de Seuil, 1994.

Lacan, Jacques. (1957–1958). *The Formations of the Unconscious*. In *The Seminar of Jacques Lacan, Book V*, translated by Russell Grigg, edited by Jacques-Alain Miller. Cambridge: Polity Press, 2017.

Lacan, Jacques. (1958a). "The Direction of the Treatment and the Principles of its Power". In *The First Complete Edition in English*, edited by Bruce Fink, pp. 489–542. London: W.W. Norton & Co., 2006.

Lacan, Jacques. (1958b). "The Signification of the Phallus". In *Écrits: The First Complete Edition in English*, edited by Bruce Fink, pp. 575–584. London: W.W. Norton & Co., 2006.

Lacan, Jacques. (1958c). "Guiding Remarks for a Congress on Female Sexuality". In *Écrits: The First Complete Edition in English*, edited by Bruce Fink, pp. 610–620. London: W.W. Norton & Co. 2006.

Lacan, Jacques. (1960). "The Subversion of the Subject and the Dialectic of Desire in the Freudian Unconscious". In *Écrits: The First Complete Edition in English*, edited by Bruce Fink, 671–702. London: W.W. Norton & Co., 2006.

Lacan, Jacques. (1962–1963). *On Anxiety*. In *The Seminar of Jacques Lacan, Book X*, translated by A. R. Price, edited by Jacques-Alain Miller. London: Polity Press, 2014.

Lacan, Jacques. (1963). *The Names-of-the-Father*. In *Television: A Challenge to the Psychoanalytic Establishment*, translated by Denis Hollier, Rosalind Krauss, Annette Michelson and Jeffrey Mehlman, edited by Joan Copjec, pp. 81–95. New York:: W.W. Norton & Co., 1999.

Lacan, Jacques. (1964). *The Four Fundamental Concepts of Psychoanalysis*. In *The Seminar of Jacques Lacan, Book XI*, translated by Alan Sheridan, edited by Jacques-Alain Miller. New York: Norton, 1998.

Lacan, Jacques. (1969). "Note on the Child". In R. Grigg (trans.), Analysis (No. 2). Melbourne Centre for Psychoanalytic Research, Deakin: Deakin Printery. 1990. Republished in *The Lacanian Review*, No. 4, 13–14, 2018.

Lacan, Jacques. (1972–1973). *On Feminine Sexuality: The Limits of Love and Knowledge*. In *The Seminar of Jacques Lacan, Book XX*, translated by Bruce Funk, edited by Jacques-Alain Miller. London: W.W. Norton and Co., 1999.

Lynn, David and Vaillant, George. (1998). "Anonymity, Neutrality, and Confidentiality in the Actual Methods of Sigmund Freud: A Review of 43 Cases, 1907–1939". *The American Journal of Psychiatry*, 155(2), 163–171.

Pfeiffer, E. (ed.). (1972). *Sigmund Freud and Lou Andreas-Salomé Letters*. New York: Harcourt, Brace & Jovanovich.

Pommier, Gérard. (2000). "Existe-t-il une distribution logique des homosexualités?" *La Clinique Lacanienne 4: Les Homosexualités*, pp. 73–99.

Rich, Adrienne. (1986). "Compulsory Heterosexuality and the Lesbian Continuum". In *Blood, Bread, and Poetry: Selected Prose, 1979–1985*. New York: Norton.

Rieder, Ines and Voigt, Diana. (2019) *The Story of Sidonie C.: Freud's Famous "Case of Female Homosexuality"*, translated by Jill Hannum and Ines Rieder. Budapest: Helena History Press.

Roudinesco, Elisabeth. (1997). *Jacques Lacan*, translated by B. Bray. New York: Columbia University Press.

Shapira, Michal. (2023). *Sigmund Freud and His Patient Margarethe Csonka: A Case of Homosexuality in a Woman in Modern Vienna*. New York: Routledge.

Spitz, René. (1945). "Hospitalism: An Inquiry into the Genesis of Psychiatric Conditions in Early Childhood". *The Psychoanalytic Study of the Child*, 1: 53–74.

Spitz, René. (1966). *The First Year of Life: A Psychological Study of Normal and Deviant Object Relations*. New York: International Universities Press.

Weiss, Eduardo. (1970). *Sigmund Freud as a Consultant: Recollections of a Pioneer in Psychoanalysis*. New York: Intercontinental Medical Book.

LITTLE HANS

Analysis of a Phobia in
a Five-Year-Old Boy

HERBERT GRAF

Born 10 April 1903, Vienna
Died 5 April 1973, Geneva

Now it will always be like this...

Freud, Sigmund. (1909). "Analysis of a Phobia in
a Five-Year-Old Boy". In *The Standard Edition of the
Complete Psychological Works of Sigmund Freud*, translated
by James Strachey, vol. 10, pp. 3–149. London: Hogarth, 1955.

DOI: 10.4324/9781032663746-8

Horses for Courses

Psychoanalysis and a Small Boy

Carol Owens

According to psychoanalytic scholarship, the case of Little Hans has entered the annals of psychoanalysis as a paradigmatic exemplar illustrating Freud's concept of the castration complex, the nosological category of anxiety hysteria, and an aetiological theory of phobias. In what follows, I will consider what psychoanalysis has claimed to learn, and could learn yet, from the case of Little Hans. I will focus on the case as it is reported in Freud's account and then look to the elaboration of the analysis of the case performed by Lacan in his fourth seminar, *The Object Relation* (Lacan [1956–1957] 2020). Later I will examine some of Darian Leader's remarks from his re-examination of the case following his analysis of the derestricted material (Leader, 2021). According to Freud (from the last page of his discussion of the case), he "learnt nothing new ... nothing that I had not already been able to discover ... from other patients analysed at a more advanced age" (Freud [1909], 147). What Freud already had discovered in older patients was that their neuroses could be traced back to the same infantile complexes that were revealed behind Hans's phobia. I will start off by looking at what Freud learnt, or rather what he didn't learn from Hans; that is, we will see what Freud already knew but found – to his delight – in Hans.

Freud's Nonsense

Some 80 pages or so of the case are given over to what is called the "Case History and Analysis" of Hans's "nervous disorder", so named by Max Graf, his father, or his "nonsense", so named by Freud; his non-sense, neither making sense for Hans or his father, or for Freud. The case history is an odd document: part reported dialogue between Max and Herbert Graf, part anecdotal report from Max to Freud, part surmising and asides from Freud about what is going on in and between the reports, some drawings of giraffes, horses, and a crude map of the street where the Grafs lived in Vienna.

What is happening with Hans in January 1908? The little boy is afraid that a horse will bite him in the street, and this seems to be connected with a fear of large penises, which Max Graf surmises may be related to an earlier observation of Hans that horses have large penises, and that his mother – being as big as a

DOI: 10.4324/9781032663746-9

horse – must have a horse-size widdler. Max wonders then, could *this all be about Hans's mother*? A good question, as it turns out. But Freud rather pushes away Max's hypothesis, declaring just two pages into this account that it is not our business to understand a case at once (p. 22). Just two pages later, however, Freud contradicts this early bit of counsel addressed to his readers and seizing on the early material at his disposal as being "amply sufficient for getting our bearings" and insisting now that "no moment of time is so favourable for the understanding of a case as the initial stage" (p. 24). Such paradoxical instructions – not to try to understand at once and to understand right at the beginning – seems like, dare I say it, a bit of nonsense.

What Freud Learns

Indeed, Freud finds quite a lot in Hans's symptom despite his saying at the end that he learns nothing new. In particular, he is able to develop a theory about phobia formation, he is able to formulate a new nosological category – the anxiety-hysterias – and he is able to place castration and the Oedipus complex as central to the origin of the anxiety neuroses.

In the second section of the "case history", in the space of just two pages, Freud sets down in chronological order the events that constitute the "beginning of Hans' anxiety and his phobia" (p. 24) and in short what happened to Hans one winter morning that transformed a previously "cheerful, good-natured and lively little boy" into a neurotically anxious child (p. 6). He summarises:

> The disorder set in with thoughts that were at the same time fearful and tender, and then followed an anxiety dream on the subject of losing his mother and so not being able to coax with her any more. His affection for his mother must therefore have become enormously intensified. This was the fundamental phenomenon in his condition … It was this increased affection for his mother which turned suddenly into anxiety—which, as we should say, succumbed to repression.
>
> (pp. 24–25)

Now this is a crucial turning point for the development and elaboration of a new piece of metapsychology for Freud. For it is precisely this bit of libido, changed into anxiety, that expresses itself in the phobia that a white horse will bite him.

Freud insists that "the horse must be his father" (p. 123) and that the fear of horses is a displaced fear of his father. Hans was afraid of his father, Freud argues, because "he himself nourished jealous and hostile wishes against him" (p. 123). This theory of anxiety, linked to the problem of libido, was a central aspect of Freud's earliest model of repression, the Oedipus complex, and the infantile neuroses (Midgeley 2006; Rodriguez 2019). At the same time, this theory of anxiety slides into the newly coined category anxiety-hysteria. Unlike conversion hysteria, the pathogenic material under repression is not converted into a somatic event but rather is set free in the shape of an anxiety or phobia. In fact, as Freud puts it: an anxiety-hysteria tends to develop more and more into a "phobia". In the end. the patient may have got rid of all his anxiety, "but only at the price of subjecting himself to all kinds of inhibitions and restrictions" (Freud 1909, 116–117).

The phobia is therefore formed as a consequence of the mind constantly at work psychically binding the anxiety which has become liberated (Compton 1992, 215; Rodriguez 2019). As the liberated anxiety cannot retransform into libido or establish any contact with the complexes which are the source of the libido, every subsequent occasion that can produce (we might say nowadays "trigger") anxiety is obstructed in the form of inhibitions and prohibitions, and defensive structures that appear in the form of phobias.

Freud Re-Reading Little Hans

Freud returned several times to the case of Hans. In 1913, in his paper "Totem and Taboo", he discusses the function of totemism in childhood and makes a few remarks about Hans. Here his emphasis is upon the elevation of the animal in an animal phobia to the status of a totem, or substitute for the child's father. He says:

> the new fact that we have learnt from the analysis of 'little Hans' – a fact with an important bearing upon totemism – is that in such circumstances children displace some of their feelings from their father on to an animal.
>
> (Freud 1913, 129)

But by all accounts, it is his return to the case in his 1926 work, "Inhibitions, Symptoms and Anxiety", in which he re-formulates the aetiological link between anxiety and symptom that has the most far-reaching effects (Freud 1926). Freud moves away from the notion of anxiety as the symptomatic manifestation of unsatisfied libido and moves towards a concept of anxiety, according to which anxiety operates as a signal that sets in motion defensive operations and the constitution of symptoms (e.g., Midgeley 2006; Rodriguez 2019). Freud's first theory of anxiety outlined in the 1909 case study explains that when libidinal longings come up against the threat of castration, a process of repression leads to the unacceptable wish becoming unconscious and the loving feelings being transformed into anxiety. In "Inhibitions, Symptoms and Anxiety", the theory is revised. As he puts it: "further investigation shows that what he was suffering from was not a vague fear of horses but a quite definite apprehension that a horse was going to bite him" (Freud 1926, 101). Rereading, or rather re-investigating the case of Little Hans as Freud describes his activity in 1926, he will arrive at the revolutionary idea that "it was anxiety which produced repression and not, as I formerly believed, repression that produced anxiety" (pp. 108–109). Interestingly it will be his idea from "Totem and Taboo" that the tendency to displace feelings of fear from the father onto an animal will allow him to make the theoretical and conceptual leap and claim that the anxiety felt in animal phobias is the untransformed fear of castration. This, Freud says here, is a "realistic fear", a fear of a danger which "was actually impending or was judged to be a real one" (p. 108). In a classic illustration of the title of his essay, Freud proposes that: "Little Hans's unaccountable fear of horses was the *symptom* and his inability to go out into the streets was an *inhibition*, a restriction which his ego had imposed on itself so as not to arouse the *anxiety*-symptom" (p. 101, emphasis added).

Thus reformulated, the fear of being castrated is seen by the ego as a danger which releases a "signal anxiety". Hans's Oedipal murderous impulses toward his father (that he should fall down and hurt himself just as the horse had done) is repressed and re-emerges as the more acceptable but nonetheless phobic fear of being bitten by a horse (Compton 1992, 222; Midgeley 2006, 542).

And Now for Something Completely Different, or What Lacan Learns

I'll begin with some remarks of Lacan's from his Geneva lecture on the symptom from 1975. He says:

> If you study the case of Little Hans closely, you will see that what appears there is what he calls his *Wiwimacher*, because he doesn't know how to call it anything else, is introduced into his circuit … One only needs to know that with certain beings, whatever they are called, the encounter with their own erection is not at all autoerotic. It is the most hetero thing there is. They ask themselves, 'But what is this?' And they wonder about it so much that this poor Little Hans thinks of nothing else and incarnates it in the most external of all objects, namely in this horse that paws the ground, that kicks, rolls over and falls to the ground. This horse that comes and goes, that has a certain way of drawing a cart along the quay, is for him the most exemplary thing of everything he is caught up in, but that he understands absolutely nothing of, owing to the fact, to be sure, that he has a certain type of mother and a certain type of father. His symptom is the expression, the meaning of this rejection … The enjoyment that has resulted from this Wiwimacher is alien to him – so much so that it is at the root of his phobia. 'Phobia' means he has got the wind up.
>
> (Lacan [1975] 1989, 15–16)

I find it interesting that, for Lacan, so late in his career, just six years before his death, he is still finding something from the case of Little Hans that is worthy of extraction to support his theories of the symptom but also how he emphasises the part that the parent's desire for the child has in the construction of the symptom. As he puts it:

> Parents mould the subject in this function that I call *symbolism*. Strictly speaking this means, not that the child is in any way the basis of a symbol, but that

the way in which a mode of speaking has been instilled in him can only bear the
mark of the mode in which his parents have accepted him. I well know that this
can have all sorts of variations, and fortunes.

(Lacan [1975] 1989, 13, emphasis in original)

Back some 20 years, in his fourth seminar from the year on the object relation,
Lacan ([1956–1957] 2022) addresses the core of what makes the case of Hans
foundational for psychoanalysis and at the same time proposes an upgrade of key
psychoanalytic concepts and of their formative effects for the human subject. So
we will see right away that in the same way that Hans served an important function for Freud, offering proof and support of his theories on infantile sexuality, the
castration and Oedipus complexes, and the advancement of a theory of anxiety, so
too will Lacan deploy the lessons of Little Hans in such a way as to offer a new take
on the castration and Oedipus complexes as well as a new aetiology of phobias,
and a conceptual framework to identify the family's historical constellations that
determine these neurotic formations.

So we will begin first with Lacan's reversal of the terms that constitute the phobia: if for Freud, the horse was a substitute for the threatening father, for Lacan, the
horse is first of all posed as a substitute for the devouring mother. Lacan begins his
analysis of Hans's phobia by saying that he wants to give due consideration to the
fundamental situation with regard to the child's phallus in relation to the mother.
Lacan's seminars of the 1950s are filled with reference to the phallus, which behaves differently according to what he is thinking about at the time. I will not go
into every twist and turn along the highways and byways of Lacan's use of the
phallus, restricting the discussion here to only a limited number. Instead, I refer you
to what is an excellent essay on the phallus and its permutations in Lacan's work
during these years by Olga Cox Cameron (2021).

In Seminar IV, the phallus functions as one of the three elements in the imaginary triangle that constitutes the preoedipal phase. It is an imaginary object that
circulates between mother and child, with the mother desiring it and the child seeking to satisfy her desire by identifying with the phallus. In the Oedipus complex,
the father intervenes as a fourth term by castrating the child, that is, by prohibiting
the child's identification as the mother's phallus, what she lacks.

According to Lacan, in the beginning, there is a child and another subject (the
mOther), one who is already installed in the symbolic order, and hence "castrated".
She is a being who is divided and marked with double lack: symbolic and imaginary. Because she is a *woman* she is *deprived* of what Lacan calls the symbolic
phallus. Her *minus* of phallus is at the same time an inscription in the symbolic
order as presence. Because she is a *castrated subject*, she desires the phallus that
she is missing, in Lacanian terms, the imaginary phallus. This is not a desire that
can be sated as it is metonymic. But she may very well attempt to sate it with her
child. In this way, her own search for the phallus may be calmed somewhat through
the child while at the same time the child cannot match up to the missing phallus,
which remains irreducible in the mother. At the precise moment when the subject

discovers that this imaginary phallus is lacking to the mother, they can find themselves engaged in coming to be a substitute for it.

In so far as the child is engaged with this psychical operation, bringing in herself or himself and their own lack to fulfil this specific lack in the mother, it dawns on the child that no satisfaction by any real object can match the mother's lack, and the inevitable experience of inadequacy, impotence and anxiety that will accompany the boy's not measuring up to the task engages him in a game of lure/deception and trickery with the mother. Ultimately, he can be led to the shattering conclusion that nothing he has, or is, will be enough for the mother. The emergence of the horse that bites in the case of Little Hans is, Lacan argues – because of regression on the oral-sadistic plane – what he calls the *real* mother, biting and devouring ([1956–1957] 2022, 358, 371). Tying Little Hans to his new theorising, he puts it this way:

> *the horse bites*, that is to say – *Since I can no longer satisfy mother at all, she will take satisfaction, just as I did when she did not satisfy me at all, biting me as I bit her, for this is my last line of recourse when I cannot be sure of her love.*
> (p. 350, italics in original)

The bite is, on the one hand, linked to the surging of something that happens each time the mother's love is lacking but it is also linked to the excitement Hans experiences in his own penis, as he describes it: "it bites him" (Freud 1909, 30, f1). The phobia thus displaces anxiety from the biting mother (and perhaps indeed away from the biting penis) onto the biting horse. Because of this reasoning Lacan says that all phobic objects in childhood are signifiers belonging to the same genre: lions, tigers and bears, for example. And it is for this reason that some phobic objects from childhood transmute into fetish objects, having had their origin in a childhood pleasure/*jouissance*. Indeed, it is even thinkable that behind the phobia of the biting horse there is the original phobic object as displaced, that is to say, the biting penis, the "widdler", the thing that gives pleasure but becomes a source of anxiety.

As such, according to Lacan's theorising at this time, it is an accident of development or a kind of historic incident that damages the links of the mother-child relation with regard to the phallus, which is what the woman lacks and the child discovers as lacking in the mother. When the harnessing of these three objects is broken, there is more than one solution possible. One of these possible outcomes is that the father intervenes as a fourth term and paves the way towards Oedipus via his threat of castration and a second privation of the mother, a symbolic operation that allows the child to renounce being the imaginary phallus for the mother. When this path is not available, as in the case of Little Hans whose "*Vatti*" (as regarded by both Freud and Lacan) is a *Daddy* who is too kind to be sufficiently menacing, when there is no exit from the game of the lure – as Lacan says later in the seminar – a phobia constitutes a call to rescue. This is why Lacan formulates the phobia as the signifier in the place of the missing father ([1956–1957] 2022, 220).

This idea that the phobia is a signifier in the place of the missing father is linked to the theorisation of the paternal metaphor which we will look at next.

Little Hans and the Paternal Metaphor

Quite early on in Seminar IV Lacan says, "For the mother, there is nearly always this requirement of the phallus on the side of the child. The child symbolises, sometimes more, sometimes less, the phallus" ([1956–1957] 2022, 48). Hans, who experiences himself to be identified with the imaginary phallus, is someone who is subjected to great anxiety. Although we see how Hans made attempts to separate from his mother, for example, in his plan to go and sleep with his friend, Mariedl, these plans were thwarted, and so his anxiety persisted. Freud, if you recall, mistakenly tried to convince Hans that his father was not angry with him for being in love with his mother. But Freud's intervention was based on the assumption that Hans's anxiety was rooted in a fear of castration rather than a wish for it. Here's Lacan's rather withering comment, on how Olga, Hans's mother, kept him close:

> Everything in the mother's conduct with little Hans, whom she literally drags around with her everywhere, from the WC to her bed, clearly indicates that the child is an absolutely indispensable appendage for her. Hans's mother, of whom Freud is very fond, to whom Freud had previously been *of assistance*, this *excellent and devoted mother*, *sehr besorgte*, and pretty to boot, still finds the wherewithal to take off her knickers in front of her child.
>
> (Lacan [1956–1957] 2022, 235)

Lacan makes the point that Hans's father should have intervened, separating the child from his mother by being convincingly angry, jealous, or authoritative in his prohibition of the mother-child over-proximity. It is in making just that point that Lacan first coins the term "paternal metaphor". The paternal metaphor is what enables the child to separate from the mother's desire and successfully pass through the Oedipus complex. The metaphor's structure is that the Name (*nom*) or No (*non*)-of-the-father stands in for the mother's desire. At this point in Lacan's work, the metaphor is the structure of the symptom, in which one signifier stands in for another which is repressed. Similarly, with the installation of the paternal metaphor, the signifier which is repressed or is under the bar has to do with the mother's insatiable desire for the child, whereas the signifier above the bar is the paternal "No!" or prohibition. It is worth noting that Lacan ([1955–1956] 2020) pointed out in his seminar on the psychoses just the year before that the paternal function can be carried out by someone other than a father. Nevertheless, Lacan used the term "paternal" to indicate that in the 1950s it was most commonly the father who took on this function. The father does not even have to be especially frightening in order to help his child undergo Oedipalisation. His role as an authoritative voice that can at least sometimes change the mother's mind is what counts.

In the case of Little Hans, Lacan commented that Hans reached an impasse in trying to separate from his mother:

> He cannot get out of it [of the grip of his mother] because there is no Father. There is nothing to metaphorize his relations with his mother. To spell it right out, there is no way out of … the castration complex.
>
> ([1956–1957] 2022, 371)

As such, the phobia makes up for a deficiency in the paternal metaphor. In fact, Lacan goes on to explain that the phobia is established or written with the same formula as the paternal metaphor except that the horse is in the place of Name-of-the-Father (pp. 370–371).

The phobic object is a signifier, as Lacan wrote in his "Direction of the Treatment" paper. It can play the role of "an all-purpose signifier to make up for [*suppléer*] the Other's lack" (Lacan 1958 [2006], 510). The horse for Little Hans does the work of signification, of plugging up the anxiety-provoking lack in the Other; the emergence of which is far more dreadful than the fear that is localised by the phobia. For Lacan, Hans's phobia was an attempt, however insufficient, to establish an order that resembled the normative order of the law of castration.

Who Are You, Herbert Graf?

Judith Chused puts it to us, so:

> [W]hat if Little Hans were here today, in an analyst's office in the twenty-first century, overstimulated, his inconsistent mothering partly compensated for by an attentive, caring father, presenting a family history of affective disorders and symptoms that would eventually reveal him to be in strong conflict over erotic longings and destructive impulses directed at both parents?
>
> (Chused 2007, 773)

In his "Re-reading Little Hans" paper, Darian Leader begins with the remark that first Max Graf, then Freud, understand Hans's phobia from within an Oedipal framework in terms of a longing for the mother, and parricidal wishes and rivalry towards the father (Leader 2021). Leader asks whether in our own prefabricated readings of the case we do not run the risk of a similar interpretative bias, despite the derestriction of papers and letters which reveal a rather different family set-up than the otherwise idyllic one depicted in the case history. He questions whether any psychoanalyst has ever encountered a child who lived in a preoedipal paradise with its mother. Moreover, he challenges the idea that the first three and a half years of Hans's life were otherwise so uneventful, only characterised by a phallic hide and seek with the mother, and undisturbed by all the forces that child analysts and researchers have shown to be so ubiquitous in early life. Leader says we tend to repeat our clearly inadequate explanations and almost wilfully ignore everything that might suggest a different approach to the case.

In Leader's own re-evaluation of the case, he comments positively on Lacan's analyses of the case, clearly finding in Lacan's "more subtle" investigation, especially his application of the Lévi-Straussian idea of the formulation of myth both useful and productive. The notion of the development of successive permutations of an initial problem in order to generate different forms of the impossibility of a solution was deployed by Lacan in order to understand what function the phobia in its various permutations served at given moments of the phobia. Indeed, Lacan's attention to the signifiers at work in the case are valued by Leader as indicating important developments. Take, for example, the noting of the two different terms for the plumber fantasies – first, *Der Klempner* and, second, *Der Installateur*. Each concerns a different act taking place and by very different kinds of agents; whereas the plumber is only concerned with Hans's waterworks, the installer is someone who fixes things, puts things right, installs things. Next Leader moves on to a contemplation of the recently surfaced biographical material, and sharpening his analytic tools, he sets out some important points.

We do need to bear in mind though what case we are dealing with here, when we're reading about Herbert, not Hans. In fact, the title of Leader's paper is a bit of a misnomer, for we are not exactly re-reading Little Hans but rather following a very comprehensive assemblage of the derestricted material in order to retroactively understand the bigger picture of the early life of Herbert Graf. As such, I think the new material behaves rather like a palimpsest. There is the case of Little Hans, and then there is the real-life material belonging to Herbert Graf. It goes on, there are the scores and scores of scholarly articles on Freud's analysis of Hans; and then many drawing on Lacan's upgrade in his fourth seminar. Now there are a good number of articles re-reading Hans via the derestricted material.

So no, there was no mother and child paradise for Herbert. Rather there were frequent and violent rows between the parents, and frequent threats of abandonment and beating of Herbert and actual frequent beating of his infant sister. Not only was Herbert's mother violent, aggressive and by these new accounts deeply psychologically unwell, she had little or no interest in her children. Difficult to imagine then is Herbert's phallic value for Olga, says Leader. What then to make of the idea so important to Freud that Herbert clung to Olga in his little Oedipus role? Well, Leader conjectures that Herbert may very well have sought her out and clung to her in order to keep both himself and his mother safe; that perhaps he could manage to stop her leaving, abandoning them/him, that perhaps it was his fault she would leave? Indeed, the same logic helps Leader to understand why Herbert tried to get into his parent's bed, or room. Since Olga became distressed – *erupted* – following any form of sexual advance by Max, perhaps Herbert jumped in to try to prevent her becoming so distraught. Leader says we could imagine a kind of hypervigilance in this boy and a terrible fear of his parents separating – a threat that was continually present throughout his childhood. Given his state of anxiety hypothesised in this account, Leader proposes that we can read Herbert's apparent zeal for masturbation less as an erotic link to his mother and more as self-consolation or comfort as well as a kind of reassuring act of separation from his mother. Leader then goes on to make a very astute and original set of observations which in fact can be really considered as re-reading Little Hans, as in, re-reading the actual case material and finding something new. He points out that neither Freud nor Lacan make enough, actually hardly anything at all, of Hans's concerns about loss and departure. Leader reads these concerns in the references Hans makes to horses drawing carts that contain a body as a possible reference to a funeral carriage rather than the representation of pregnancy that Freud makes of it, and he does a lot of this by following the signifiers in the case material itself.

But indeed, a prevailing element in the various re-readings of Little Hans is hearing how the child's speech is heard by his parents and by Freud. How it is heard, how it is misheard, how some elements are never singled out for reflection while others are heavily foregrounded. A simple little example. We are told that when Hans was three and a half, his mother threatens that a doctor will come and cut off his widdler if he continues to put his hand on it. "Then what'll you widdle with?" she asks (Freud 1909, 8). He replies: "With my bottom" (p. 35). Here we have a fascinating insight into this 3-year-old's idea that it could be possible to swap out his penis for his bottom, that the two things are interchangeable at the level of function for Little Hans. This early little bit of 3-year-old wisdom actually can be seen to be a precursor to the installer fantasy of his 5-year-old mind; an installer guy will come and swap out his widdler and his behind for bigger ones. If the installer fantasy is taken as the proof that Hans accepts castration, surely, we can see that even at three years of age and long before all of the discussions and conversations around his widdler have taken place that Hans already knows that some things might have to be given up but that something else might do the job equally well.

Listening to Little Hans, trying to listen to him considering the heavy editing and censoring that have taken place, it seems to me that in the careful selection of material by first Max and then by Freud of what makes it into the case write-up, we only glimpse the young child's babbling, as Lacan calls it, when Max lets him babble on and we know that that's for a reason.

I would say, and I know that Kristen Hennessy agrees with me here, that there is no doubt that what we now know about the early childhood of Herbert Graf makes it impossible to just read the Little Hans case in the ways that either Freud or Lacan did. But I guess what I want to emphasise is that with or without access to the derestricted material, it behoves us to re-read all of the Freud case studies with a different approach (what this volume attempts to do, in fact). It seems to me that our different approaches will always reflect – actually *ought to* reflect – our own situated investments with the case. As with Freud and Lacan, when we read Little Hans, we also read from our own invested positions. As it happens, my own investment is naturally inclined to discerning the adolescent voice, the one we hear of big Hans, Herbert, when he returns to visit Freud in 1922, this is because my own clinical work is for the most part a clinic of adolescence.

There is a neat little warning in the case of Little Hans which we can take seriously for our clinical work. It goes like this: "Hey Analyst! Don't sit down with a young person in a room and curate their babblings to lead that speech to the place you think it should be headed. You might have to hear them say to you: I say, all of this is only a joke!" In fact, I did hear this once but thankfully it was a remark made about a former therapist of a 13-year-old girl I was working with! As in, the therapist was a joke! Why? Because everything the young person told her about led to a series of questions and interrogations for further details; eventually the young client had spun a whole story into being, ludicrous and terrifying, and when the therapist was on the edge of her seat, practically on speed dial for the police and the social workers, the young client collapsed in giggles; it was all a joke, it was all just a joke. And that was the end of that. So when she came to see me, she told me this tale of her "airheaded" therapist. *Her* expression. I took note.

All going well, every 5-year-old grows up and becomes a 19-year-old adolescent. The strapping youth who visits Freud in 1922 declares himself to be perfectly well (that is, no harm done by the analysis or its publication which Freud might have been worried about, judging by the weight Freud gives to this declaration of good mental health), suffering from no inhibitions or troubles. However, he lived alone, his parents had divorced, and he was estranged from his young sister. All of this Freud takes at face value, even though this pretty little paragraph really tells us very little about *Big Hans*! In the Eissler interview conducted in 1959 with Herbert Graf, it is so clear that meeting Freud in 1922 was a real buzz for him and showing how highly he held Freud in his esteem, comparing him to Sophocles but also stressing how paternal he found him. Of course, he couldn't remember any detail of the so-called treatment, a point that Freud is keen to theorise as a harmless bit of amnesia after a satisfactory analysis. Later in his life, Herbert Graf at 55 years of age can only remember feeling afraid to leave the house during a certain time of his life, and of horses falling, and of fire. But in a way, this postscript only reveals that Herbert Graf has (1) forgotten the events of his 5-year-old life, and (2) he is impressed with Freud. But what we don't know anything about, and sadly never will, is why Herbert met with Freud then. What did he want to say? What might he have said if Freud wasn't so keen to wrap it all up and show how Herbert finding himself published as *the Little Hans* didn't do him any harm?

References

Chused, Judith F. (2007). "Little Hans 'Analyzed' in the Twenty-First Century". *Journal of the American Psychoanalytic Association* 55, 767–778.

Compton, Alan. (1992). "The Psychoanalytic View of Phobias: Part: Freud's Theory of Phobia and Anxiety". *Psychoanalytic Quarterly* 61, 206–229.

Cox Cameron, Olga. (2021). "The Phallus of the Fifties: Those Years of 'Tranquil Possession'". In *Studying Lacan's Seminar VI: Dream, Symptom, and the Collapse of Subjectivity*, edited by Olga Cox Cameron and Carol Owens. London: Routledge.

Freud, Sigmund. (1909). "Analysis of a Phobia in a Five-Year-Old Boy". In *The Standard Edition of the Complete Psychological Works of Sigmund Freud*, translated by James Strachey, vol. 10, pp. 3–149. London: Hogarth, 1955.

Freud, Sigmund. (1913). "Totem and Taboo". In *The Standard Edition of the Complete Psychological Works of Sigmund Freud*, translated by James Strachey, vol. 13, pp. 1–164. London: Hogarth, 1955.

Freud, Sigmund. (1926). "Inhibitions, Symptoms and Anxiety". In *The Standard Edition of the Complete Psychological Works of Sigmund Freud*, translated by James Strachey, vol. 20, pp. 77–178. London: Hogarth, 1955.

Lacan, Jacques. (1955–1956). *The Psychoses*. In *The Seminar of Jacques Lacan, Book III*, translated by Russell Grigg, edited by Jacques-Alain Miller. London: Polity Press, 2020.

Lacan, Jacques. (1956–1957). *The Object Relation*. In *The Seminar of Jacques Lacan, Book IV*, translated by Adrian Price, edited by Jacques-Alain Miller. London: Routledge, 2022.

Lacan, Jacques. (1958). "The Direction of the Treatment and the Principles of its Power". In *Écrits: The First Complete Edition in English*, translated by Bruce Fink. New York: W.W. Norton and Company, 2006.

Lacan, Jacques. (1975). "Geneva Lecture on the Symptom", translated by Russell Grigg. *Analysis* 1(7), 1989.

Leader, Darian. (2021). "Rereading Little Hans". Centre for Freudian Analysis and Research. Available at: https://jcfar.org.uk/jcfar-bookshop/digital-editions/rereading-little-hans/.

Midgeley, Nicholas. (2006). "Re-Reading 'Little Hans': Freud's Case Study and the Question of Competing Paradigms in Psychoanalysis". *Journal of the American Psychoanalytic Association* 54(2), 537–559.

Rodriguez, Leonardo. (2019). "The Lessons of Little Hans". In *Studying Lacan's Seminars IV and V: From Lack to Desire*, edited by Carol Owens and Nadezhda Almqvist. London: Routledge.

Chapter 6

Little Hans in Context

Kristen Hennessy

Introduction

We all know Freud's Little Hans. He is that happy child from a happy family who is being raised in an atmosphere described by Freud as being as free of coercion as possible (Freud 1909, 6). To put it more precisely, the parents had agreed that "in bringing up their first child they would use no more coercion than might be absolutely necessary" (p. 6). There's a nuance in this passage which suggests that Freud had made them promise that. Hans develops a phobia in the context of his mother's over-investment in his penis and his father's ineffective efforts to place limits on the mother and child. This little boy, his fear of horses, and unending questions about widdlers, teach us valuable lessons about phobia, but also about sexuality in childhood and childhood neurosis.

Then, there is also Herbert Graf, the child whose material was written up as Little Hans. As we will see, Herbert's family situation was not exactly free of strife, nor was Herbert's childhood carefree by any stretch of the imagination. At the time of publication, the case was presented with very little information about the child. This was partly because Freud was endeavouring to demonstrate with this account that sexuality operates this way for normal, healthy children, and the details of a messy family system would only detract from this mission. It is also likely that the omission of the details was for other reasons which I will discuss later.

This chapter will outline the child's family history, with an ear to what this adds to our understanding of the case. I will argue that understanding Little Hans with the added lens of Herbert Graf's history allows us to understand the child's specific predicament, to whom his symptoms are addressed and why. In his article, "Rereading Little Hans," Darian Leader (2021) challenges us to take up the information about the child's biography in our interpretations of this case. There is never a penultimate interpretation, and this chapter seeks to add to, not replace, other interpretations of this case.

Herbert Graf

As any analyst can attest, there is no *objective* recounting of a life. Nevertheless, the events of a life are notable and are certainly fodder for analysis. No analysis is complete without delving into the subject's history, and doing so in its specificity,

DOI: 10.4324/9781032663746-10

its singularity. The history must be articulated during the course of an analysis. Herbert's story begins, as all stories do, well before his birth.

His mother, Olga Hönig, had her own particularly painful childhood in which her father died in her infancy, her brothers each committed suicide, and her sister (who had infantile paralysis) attempted suicide (Borch-Jacobsen 2021, 89). At 19 years old, Olga went into analysis with Freud. Olga's mother paid for this analysis until Olga made accusations of sexual abuse against her brothers. Freud, according to Borch-Jakobson, continued to treat her for free, an offer she initially accepted (p. 89). She began to date Max, Herbert's father, and spoke with him about her analysis with Freud. The tales of analysis apparently intrigued Max who decided he needed to meet this Freud guy. Freud became his confidante and he ultimately asked Freud if they should marry. "By all means marry her. You will have fun." Yet fun, Max later said, "we did not have" (Graf 1952, 75). Olga ultimately, angrily, broke off her analysis with Freud, speaking negatively of him thenceforth, a situation that seems to have been exacerbated by his ongoing involvement in her life.

The marriage was troubled, and Max returned to Freud who advised having a baby, though Olga was not interested in becoming a mother. But Freud's word prevailed. After a miscarriage, Herbert was born. This was, as we might predict, not the end of the trouble (has anyone ever seen marital problems resolved via the birth of a child?).

I have discovered less with regard to Max's childhood. He told Kurt Eissler in an interview in 1952 that he was afraid of his father who would give him beatings, and whose brother was sent away to America, a place befitting someone who is "up to no good" (Graf 1952, 82). However, it is telling that Herbert later described his father, in his interview with Eissler, as "turning away" from unpleasant things, smiling even in the face of his wife's death, a man who did not attend his daughter's funeral after her suicide. The adult Herbert described his father as having a talent for turning bad things into positives or pushing them aside. In Max, we have a portrait of a talented musician who was interested in psychoanalysis but who nevertheless struggled to face unpleasant truths. He was a man who was interested in psychoanalysis but had not been analysed. We know that he had a strained relationship with his father and had his reasons for seeking out Freud as a paternal figure, a mentor of sorts. He was a man who could not recall why he chose his son's name (Graf 1952, 78).

Herbert was born to a mother who did not wish to be a mother, and to a father whose desire to be a father was spurred on by Freud. We hear, for example, that Olga would become violent and depressed after sexual intercourse, sometimes ripping or crumpling up Max's manuscripts, something absolutely in dialogue with the crumpled Giraffes (crumpled Grafs) (Leader 2021, 8). Herbert shared a bedroom with his parents until he was four years old (p. 10), so it is difficult to imagine that he was entirely unaware of these conflicts. Freud was actively involved in Max's decision-making as a parent, even being the one to determine that the child should be circumcised (p. 11), something we cannot overlook in terms of this child's questions about *widdlers*!

When Herbert's birth did not fix the marital conflict, Freud doubled down: he suggested yet another baby, resulting in the birth of Hannah. Accounts indicate that although Olga was not overly interested in mothering Herbert, she was utterly rejecting of the baby girl whom she is described as beating from as early as six months old. Hannah, the rejected baby, ultimately committed suicide in adulthood.

Freud never concealed that he brought Herbert a rocking horse, but Herbert's father first indicated that this horse was delivered on the child's third birthday and carried up four flights of stairs. This was before the identity of the child known as the Little Hans had been revealed. Afterwards, the case was edited to suggest that Freud delivered this on the child's fifth birthday, something that could be seen as an intervention and a celebration of the resolution of the child's phobia. Darian Leader points out that the number of flights of stairs up which Freud is said to have carried the horse is only consistent with the original narration, when the child lived as a 3-year-old. It is Freud who brings a horse into the home, of which the child later becomes afraid (p. 10). What do we make of this?

Also relevant is that at the time of the phobia, Little Hans was around his paternal grandfather who was terminally ill and, as Darien Leader points out, "when we read about the Sunday visits to Lainz to spend time with his grandmother in the garden there, the grandfather would have been in the house dying of a terminal illness" (p. 12). Once again, those with widdlers were dying!

It is not only Herbert's childhood context that has been sanitised, but his future as well. As an adult, Herbert sat down for an interview with Eissler.[1] The following is from the verbatim translation of this interview: "My mother still has complaints, saying that Freud was not good in her life, and advising my father to have children, and so forth, etc. It more or less broke up, off ultimately their marriage" (Graf 1959, 10). He commented that in adulthood he went to an analyst when struggling with his first wife, who struggled with alcoholism, and that he didn't like it at all! He stated:

I always had the feeling that this is the most wonderful thing on earth as, as a thought; as a science and everything, but it is too easily an … I mean, the hands of people to handle it often are not worthy of … handling it.

(p. 14)

As Darian Leader put it:

Likewise, the idea that Hans went on to have a successful and fruitful life is strange. As Lacanians, we are the first to question equations of social functionality with 'mental health': the fact that someone has a job, is married and has a network of social relationships is hardly a sign of the absence of internal pain or catastrophe, and we quite rightly challenge this, especially in contexts of the claims made by the cognitive therapies. Yet with Hans we all smile approvingly at his wonderful life, marked by successes in the opera world, the creation of more imaginary children that he had set as his compass in childhood.

Yet Herbert Graf did not agree with this sanitised version of his own life, and certainly had real children, facts that have been known for years and are even referenced in Graf's own published work. So it is curious that we choose to ignore this as we repeat our potted summaries of the case!

(Leader 2021, 7)

Does History Matter?

At the time that Lacan was delivering his fourth seminar, in which Little Hans figures so prominently, Lacan himself was critical of the idea that the history would add to the case:

People tell us that the *environmental image*, as they put it these days, of Hans's family circle has not been traced out sufficiently. What more do they want? It's enough to read the case – and not even between the lines – to see the father's constant and diligent presence spreading out, well, the mother is mentioned only to the extent that the father asks her whether what she has just said is accurate.

(Lacan [1956–1957] 2022, 313; original emphasis)

I believe that this added context opens up the possibility of new readings of what the little boy said, why he said it, and what was at stake. Of course, I have no way of knowing if Lacan would agree with me that these new details change everything even as they also change nothing.

The addition of the history, decades after the publication of the case that has become a piece of the Freudian canon, is, at least to my mind, reminiscent of the process of analysis itself. How often does an analysand circle the same material, the same signifiers repeatedly in an analysis only to suddenly, perhaps near the end of analysis, burst forth with a new detail of history in a manner that allows everything to shift? As any seasoned analyst can attest, there is no shortcut to this – there is no way to circumvent the circling, or to rush the arrival at the new material, even as the new material often functions as a key to the resolution of neurosis.

Why Was It Omitted?

I would further argue that Freud had his reasons for leaving out these details – he was publishing this material at the request of the father, Max, and both parents, Max and Olga, would surely read the publication. The Grafs were part of Freud's social circle and it is likely that family friends would recognise the case, even without the omitted details. Those details, if added, would entirely expose the family. Furthermore, Max was authorising Freud to speak about his descriptions of Herbert's sexuality, not the rest of the story. Anyone who has tried to anonymise a case can relate to some of Freud's problems – sometimes the details that are most relevant to a case are precisely those that are identifiable such as names, and specific details about the case that are core to expressing what happened in the case precisely because they are specific to this subject. We are often forced to either drop those details from our case histories or try to fictionalise the case in order to account for the details.

Freud was open about his motivation to show that there is something to his sexual theories, and he was also likely motivated to remove anything that would detract from that message – he was trying to show a case of a "normal" child from a "normal" family to demonstrate that children are sexual creatures even under those circumstances. As I said before, *normal* families turn out to be incredibly complex.

Significance

Just as a new piece of history or detail can drastically change our understanding of a particular case or symptom, so too does our understanding of what is going on with Little Hans change when we learn about the troubled life of Herbert Graf. I believe consideration of what we now know about the complexities of the child's actual life allows us to rethink this case and offers us a far better map for child psychoanalysis than we previously knew. Darian Leader says:

> Despite the fact that new material has been available for almost fifteen years now which forces a radical revision of our understanding, we tend to repeat our clearly inadequate explanations and almost wilfully ignore everything that might suggest a different approach to the case.
>
> (Leader 2021, 2)

The urge to conceal what we know about the complexity of the child's life puts *us* in the midst of a kind of family drama – what do we do when we discover information that does not fit with the narrative of our patriarch? Freud was motivated to edit out the impact of certain family dynamics on the child and his phobia. When we learn of information that Freud did not wish to feature, do we make space for this information, or do we ban it from speech, repress our knowledge of it?

This is precisely what we are tasked with when we work with children in the clinic: we must listen for what is impolite, what does not fit with what the referral source sometimes wishes for us to hear. We have to allow children to fill us in on the rest of the story, with what they know but are forbidden to know. We must make space for something other than the conscious narrative of adults to be spoken in the clinic.

But having the new information matters, absolutely. I'm grateful for it. Prior to this information, I must confess that I struggled to picture this child, to connect him to the children who come to my office to play and to speak, with all the mess of their family lives. Despite the complexity of the case, there was a kind of one-dimensionality to it. Things are never quite that simple. I'm aware that because I choose to treat children who are in foster care, their histories may be more extreme than some other children in terms of the severity of the distress, discord, and violence operating in the background, and yet, has anyone ever met a child, inside or outside of the clinic, whose life can be described as *carefree*?

I can picture this child, born into the midst of a confusing family drama, finding himself left the way that other children are left – to figure out the story not only of birth in general, but of their *own* birth in particular. Why do they exist, who wanted them here, how did it happen? Is there a space for them here? Does it belong to them?

For me, this new information allows Little Hans to come to life, and it changes our understanding of his symptoms, even as it does not undo or undermine previous understandings. Is this not how things go in analysis, anyhow? That the analysand is circling around the articulation of something connected to a symptom, then some new piece of history is articulated that somehow puts the symptom in a new light entirely, often finally leading to its resolution? That last piece, where the missing bit of history is finally articulated, never happens until after what seems to be endless circling.

The resolution to endless circling in analysis requires us to return to central questions: How did his father end up communicating with Freud about widdlers, horses, and Herbert? Freud had asked his adherents to bring him examples of childhood sexuality, in the service of bolstering his evidence for his psychoanalytic theories. He explains how the story of Little Hans came to his attention:

> Surely there must be a possibility of observing in children at first hand and in all the freshness of life the sexual impulses and wishes which we dig out so laboriously in adults from among their debris ... With this end in view I have for many years been urging my pupils and my friends to collect observations of the sexual life of children – the existence of which has a rule been cleverly overlooked or deliberately denied. Among the material which came into my possession as a result of these requests, the reports which were received at regular intervals about little Hans soon began to take a prominent place. His parents were both among my closest adherents, and they had agreed that in bringing up their first child they would use no more coercion than might be absolutely necessary for maintaining good behaviour.
>
> (Freud 1909, 6)

It seems that many parents, also followers of Freud, were reluctant to share the sexuality of their children with Freud for the purposes of publication. This leads to the question: what was different for Max? Why was Max comfortable sharing? It seems to me that he is both interested in propping up Freud, a man to whom he entrusts many major life decisions, and that he is interested in concealing, even to himself, the *rest* of the story of his son and his family.

What we see in this case is a little boy, Hans, who is dealing not with his mother's overwhelming fixation on him, but rather her own agoraphobia, violence, abhorrence of sexuality, and dislike of her own children. He is dealing with a father who continues to turn to a master instead of seeing himself in the role of the father. For

Max, it may have been easier to see his son's struggles with his sexuality than to acknowledge that there is more to the story. In other words, focusing on the child's Oedipal conflicts in this way effectively served to cover over what was painful for Max to face. Furthermore, Herbert's birth was supposed to fix the family, *per* Freud. Max may have been desperate to prove this substitute father right!

We see a little boy plagued by the questions of childhood: who has a widdler and who doesn't? Why? What can one do with one's widdler? Why are there limits on widdlers when touching them feels so nice? How are children born? Why are children born? To whom does a child belong, and what does it mean? All children ask these questions.

When we read the case with the knowledge of history in mind, we also see a little boy rather brilliantly propping up his father – precisely through the development of a phobia – whose successful analysis would finally prove Freud right! He waited until his father was writing to Freud about his sexuality to develop this symptom.

Freud gave Herbert a rocking horse.

Herbert gave his father a horse phobia to be given to Freud.

Note

1   Eissler's interviews have been derestricted for quite some time. The typed transcripts of the 1959 interview with Herbert can be viewed on the site of the Library of Congress website. This is in English (Graf 1959). Similarly, the typed transcript of Eissler's 1952 interview with Max Graf can be viewed on its site. This is in German up to page 68, then it continues in English from page 69, from which point the infancy of Herbert and the family relationships are discussed (Graf 1952).

References

Borch-Jacobsen, Mikkel. (2021). *Freud's Patients: A Book of Lives*. New York: Reaktion Books.

Freud, Sigmund. (1909). "Analysis of a Phobia in a Five-Year-Old Boy". In *The Standard Edition of the Complete Psychological Works of Sigmund Freud*, translated by James Strachey, vol. 10, pp. 5–149. New York: Norton, 1955.

Graf, Herbert. (1959). Interview by K. Eissler. Box R1, Sigmund Freud Papers. Sigmund Freud Collection, Manuscript Division, Library of Congress, Washington, DC. Manuscript/Mixed Material. Available at: http://hdl.loc.gov/loc.mss/ms004017.mss39990.01476.

Graf, Max. (1952). Interview by K. Eissler. Box R1, Sigmund Freud Papers. Sigmund Freud Collection, Manuscript Division, Library of Congress, Washington, DC. Manuscript/Mixed Material. Available at: http://hdl.loc.gov/loc.mss/ms004017.mss39990.01478.

Lacan, Jacques. (1956–1957). *The Object Relation*. In *The Seminar of Jacques Lacan, Book IV*, translated by Adrian Price. Cambridge: Polity, 2022.

Leader, Darian. (2021). "Rereading Little Hans". Centre for Freudian Analysis and Research. Available at: https://jcfar.org.uk/jcfar-bookshop/digital-editions/rereading-little-hans/.

THE RAT MAN

Notes Upon a Case of Obsessional Neurosis

ERNST LANZER

Born 22 January 1878, Vienna
Died 25 November 1914, on the Russian Front. Captured, presumed executed

His horror at a pleasure of his own of which he himself was unaware...

Freud, Sigmund. (1907–1908). "Addendum: Original Record of the Case". In *The Standard Edition of the Complete Psychological Works of Sigmund Freud*, edited by James Strachey, vol. 10, pp. 259–318. London: Hogarth, 1955.

Freud, Sigmund. (1909). "Notes Upon a Case of Obsessional Neurosis". In *The Standard Edition of the Complete Psychological Works of Sigmund Freud*, edited by James Strachey, vol. 10, pp. 155–249. London: Hogarth, 1955.

DOI: 10.4324/9781032663746-11

Chapter 7

What We Can Still Learn from the Rat Man

Astrid Gessert

I will highlight aspects of the Rat Man case that I consider useful to be aware of or reminded of when working today with obsessional subjects and taking a Lacanian perspective. There are many readings of Freud's case as there are many takes on Lacan's approach to obsessional neurosis, and there are many *definitions* of obsessional neurosis, including questions as to whether one should even think of obsession in terms of a structure, including those from Guy Le Gaufey in Chapter 8 in this collection. My contribution presents just one way of thinking about obsessional neurosis and the Rat Man case.

To begin, I will focus on the moment of when and how obsessional subjects may enter analysis. This happens when something is no longer working for them, when there is a danger of something getting out of control. For the sake of simplicity, when speaking about obsessional subject, I am following the tradition of referring to them as *obsessionals*, bearing in mind that this is somewhat problematic as it reduces the complexity of human subjects and obsessional neurosis to something like a reification. And when referring to "the obsessional", I am following the tradition of referring to this person as him. Obviously, I do not mean to imply that there are no obsessional women; neurosis is a question of structure, not of biological sex. Nevertheless, obsession seems to be more common in men, even today, when there have been great changes to the position of men and women since Freud, with women taking a much more active part in all aspects of life and society. Thinking about it psychoanalytically, one reason why we may encounter obsession more frequently in men may be because men can more easily imagine that they have *it*, the object that satisfies the Other, and also because the penis and the way it functions support the idea of an enjoyment that is limited and can be counted, stroke by stroke, so to speak, whereas the woman's *jouissance* can be unlimited (Silvestre 2018, 106).

Starting from this moment of when and how obsessionals enter analysis will help us to understand something about what happened before this moment, when things were still working, and the person was not suffering so much. In other words, this can help us to understand the function of the neurosis and how its compulsions and rituals enabled obsessionals to get through life up to a point without seeking any help.

DOI: 10.4324/9781032663746-12

To be clear, entry into analysis is not the same as the emergence of the neurosis. When obsessionals ask for treatment, the neurosis has long been established and they may have lived with their obsessions and rituals for a long time without being too much troubled by them. The Rat Man had told Freud that "he had suffered from obsessions ever since his childhood" (Freud 1909, 158) but it was only when he was 29 years old that he went to see Freud. Before that, he had managed without help, if not always very satisfactorily. He had been particularly bothered by *"fears* that something might happen to two people of whom he was very fond" and he told Freud that "he had wasted years … in fighting against these ideas of his, and that in this way had lost much ground in the course of his life" (p. 158). He had only just passed his final law examination (p. 255). Freud comments that in this case a complete obsessional neurosis had been established by the age of 7 (p. 162).

What we find with obsessionals who come for treatment is that at some point something has happened that actualises the motifs of the neurosis and upsets the carefully balanced system they have established and the equilibrium they may have achieved. Then they might seek help.

When working with obsessionals, I have found it useful to distinguish three moments, identified by Silvestre (2018, 104–105), that mark the entry into analysis:

1 Encounter with something overwhelming that produces intense anxiety.
2 Ineffectiveness of the symptom.
3 Constitution of somebody who is supposed to know how to manage this new upheaval.

These moments can be illustrated with the case of the Rat Man, and I think we can also find them in contemporary presentations of obsessional neuroses.

Encounter with Something Overwhelming and Intense Anxiety

For Freud's patient, the trigger that made him turn to Freud was his encounter with the cruel captain who told him about the rat punishment. This experience, as the Rat Man himself told Freud, was the immediate occasion of him going to see Freud. The Rat Man had observed that this captain was "obviously fond of cruelty" and he had "a kind of dread of him" (p. 166). When he heard the story of the torture, he "was overcome with anxiety. There was something in this story that he could not bear" (Silvestre 2018, 104). And he could hardly put it into words, evidenced by the gaps in his speech when he tried to tell this story to Freud. Freud helped him, for example, by providing the word "anus" (Freud 1909, 166).

Freud linked what the patient could not bear to a certain *pleasure*, an enjoyment he did not want to know about. This enjoyment became manifest in the patient's strange facial expression while telling the story of the rat punishment. Freud thought it was "horror at a pleasure of his own of which he himself was unaware" (pp. 166–167; see also Silvestre 2018, 104).

The patient then added with difficulty that at the moment he heard the story the idea flashed through his mind "that this was happening to a person who was very dear to me" (Freud 1909, 167). In fact, it turned out to be two persons: the lady he admired and his father, the father who was already dead at this time, having died nine years before of emphysema.

What was this enjoyment and whose enjoyment was it, and why was there anxiety? This becomes clear at the end of the treatment, in the resolution of the rat fantasy. In Freud's understanding, the story of the rat punishment had stirred up all of the patient's premature infantile repressed impulses of egoistic and sexual cruelty (p. 215). This produced anxiety; it confronted him with something out of bounds, like the father's rage – his father sometimes used to beat him, not knowing when to stop – and his own rage as a little boy against this cruel father for whom the captain and also Freud had become substitutes. This overwhelming pleasure in cruelty, cruelty towards an other, was unconscious, but it disrupted the obsessional world which he had established. It upset his equilibrium (Silvestre 2018, 104).

Lacan used the term *jouissance* for such excessive enjoyment. One way of understanding this multifaceted concept is that it is not the kind of pleasure that is regulated by the Freudian pleasure principle. It is not pleasure that is obtained and regulated by the reduction of a certain amount of tension. *Jouissance* is pleasure beyond pleasure, it is the ultimate pleasure that would be obtained when total satisfaction would be achieved by filling every lack, every hole (Lacan [1959-1960] 1992, 184). But this would be only possible through a total fusion with whatever object would fill this hole, like the return to the womb, and this is at the cost of disappearing as a separate subject. Note that incidentally in the torture the captain described, there is a hole in the pot, and the hole of the anus, into which the rats penetrate, holes to be filled by rats. And the Rat Man, in Freud's understanding, had identified himself with a rat. He could fill the hole in the Other, become the object of the Other, fuse with the Other. This ultimate pleasure of becoming whole again is both very enticing and very anxiety-inducing, an existential anxiety, the anxiety of disappearing. This is the obsessional's dilemma. There is too much enjoyment, which is traumatic because it is at the cost of one's own disappearance.

The encounter with *jouissance*, or at least with the prospect of it, does not have to be as dramatic as in the Rat Man case. It can take the form of meeting a woman who shows some interest in an obsessional person who, for example, had abstained from romantic relationships. In being confronted with an other's desire the obsessional may understand this as a demand to get out of his enclosed, self-sufficient system, to give up his position of desperately holding on to desire while making it impossible to engage with it. The obsessional shies away when being summoned to do something with desire that would not yield *jouissance* but a more limited pleasure (see Silvestre 2018, 107).

The patient may also not present immediately with overwhelming anxiety. Anxiety can be kept quiet under a coat of lethargy, of not being able to act, which is another symptom commonly found in obsessional neurosis (Vanheule 2001). It often takes the form that for every intended action, there is immediately a reason why it cannot be carried out. In one example, a man needed an operation but could not get on with it because he had nobody who would walk his dog; another was somebody who complained that they missed social contacts, but the people they meet are never from the right set, hence they are not worth speaking to.

Other moments that can unravel the obsessional's system can be events in his professional life such as a promotion, or completing a dissertation, moments that the person interprets as now having fulfilled what an Other wants from them, and they now have become what the Other wants them to be, like the Rat Man fulfilling the captain's demand: "Lieutenant A. has paid the charges for you. You must pay him back" (Freud 1909, 168). When an obsessional achieves what he longed for, when he gets close to what he really wants, he runs away (Vanheule 2001, 121). He is terrorised by the prospect of an enjoyment that is both extremely compelling and highly dangerous as becoming immersed in *jouissance* he would lose himself. By fulfilling the desire of the Other, he sees himself as completing the Other, becoming the object of the Other's enjoyment, and thereby again losing himself as a separate being. This is what he will avoid at all cost. This is why we can say, obsessionals suffer from *jouissance*, to the point of being obsessed with it (Silvestre 2018, 99).

What will bring obsessional subjects to see an analyst is an encounter with this enjoyment and the anxiety it evokes. And when they come, what they want to achieve is to be restored to their normal, obsessional self.

The second moment we can isolate that marks the entry into analysis is the failure of the symptom.

Ineffectiveness of the Symptom

To deal with the disruption of their balanced system, obsessionals will try to intensify their coping mechanisms such as their symptoms and rituals, or they will invent new ones, or both. The aim is separation from the threatening Other and the overwhelming *jouissance* that fusion with this Other would bring; there is a need to create a distance again. Separation is one of the hallmarks of obsessional neurosis, as Freud had observed when he noted that in the case of obsessional neurosis isolation is the typical defence mechanism. Traumatic experiences are not forgotten, as they are in hysteria, but become isolated so that they are "not reproduced in the ordinary processes of thought" (Freud 1926, 120; see also Verhaeghe 2018, 382–390).

In the case of the Rat Man, when he had the idea that the punishment might happen to the lady he admired and his already dead father, he tried to ward it off with his usual defensive measures and formulas: first, he used the word "aber" (but) and made a dismissive gesture. This worked to some extent to keep this idea at bay. The choice of the word "aber" was not arbitrary: The German word "aber" is pronounced "*a*ber", with the emphasis on the "a" but the patient had started to pronounce it "ab*e*r". with the emphasis on the "e". He explained to Freud that emphasising the end of the word gave him more protection from the intrusion of some foreign element which he so much dreaded. It is an example of a strategy to create distance, to keep things apart (Freud 1909, 224).

Another attempt at separation that Freud observed with this patient was the loss of his glasses at the spot where the captain had told the story and where the intrusive thoughts occurred (p. 165). The Rat Man could easily have found the glasses, but he did not go and look for them, instead he asked his optician in Vienna to send a new pair. For him, the look, the gaze, the scopic drive is both exciting and terrorising, manifested in the urge he felt as a boy to see women naked (pp. 160–162). So it is not by coincidence that he lost his glasses and did not go to find them. It is safer not to see, to stay away from the object of the drive (Melman 2018, 86). In Freud's understanding, "looking took the place of touching", touching and looking establish contiguity and this is what the obsessional tries to avoid as he is bound on isolation and separation (Freud 1909, 309; Mahony 2007, 96).

When the captain handed him the parcel with his new glasses a day and a half later and asked him to reimburse Lieutenant A., the Rat Man developed a new symptom: he knew that it was not Lieutenant A. who had paid for the parcel, but nevertheless he felt compelled to pay back the money to A., to somebody to whom he did not owe it. The scenario he set up is impossible and it failed in the function of pacifying what has been stirred up; this was the demand of an Other for *jouissance*, which became re-evoked by the captain's demand that he pay back the money to A. With this, there is no chance that he can "return to his tranquil world … and anxiety persists" (Silvestre 2018, 105). The gist of the symptom is as follows: he made, knowingly, an oath about paying a debt that could not be fulfilled and then, while trying to fulfil it, did at the same time everything to stop him from fulfilling it as when he took the train to Vienna and at every stop wondered if he should return to make the payment, but he didn't return.

Even after he had sent the money to the post office with the help of his friend, his doubts flared up again: He decided to see a doctor who would write him a certificate to say it was necessary to pay the money back to Lieutenant A., so that Lieutenant A. would understand and accept the money. At this moment, he found a book by Freud and went to see him. But there he did not ask for a certificate, he asked to be freed of his obsessions (Freud 1909, 173).

Another example of the ineffectiveness of symptoms are cases when obsessionals' strategies of procrastination, of "not acting" turn into an almost lethal lethargy, so that they can no longer function adequately to keep their lives together. They suffer and then they may turn to someone for help. With this we come to the third moment that marks the entry into analysis.

Constitution of Somebody Who Knows: What Lacan Called the Subject-Supposed-to-Know

When the Rat Man picked up a book by Freud in a friend's house, *The Psychopathology of Everyday Life*, the verbal associations Freud described in this book reminded him of his own "thought-work" (*Gedankenarbeit*). He thought now that there was somebody who was knowledgeable and who could understand what was happening to him, someone "who gives the impression of being able to do something about it" (Silvestre 2018, 105). So, he went to see Freud.

With these three moments we have a passage from anxiety that is evoked by an enjoyment that is about to get out of control, to a symptom that was meant to exert this control but failed, to establishing somebody who is supposed to know what to do about this (Silvestre 2018, 105).

Transference and Treatment

When entering into a relationship with the analyst as Other, obsessionals will enact their usual patterns and dilemmas they have established in relation to the Other: they give just enough to keep the Other happy so that the Other will not reveal any desire, while they retain their own unconscious desire and enjoyment. For instance, Freud (1907–1908) had noted in the eighth session (October 20, 1907), that "the lady still remains most mysterious". so he had asked the patient to bring a photo of her. In the next session, he noted (from his case notes, October 11, 1907):

> Violent struggle, bad day. Resistance, because I requested him yesterday to bring a photograph of the lady with him—i.e. to give up his reticence about her. Conflict as to whether he should abandon the treatment or surrender his secrets.
> (Freud 1907–1908, 260)

While patients may give their analysts what they think will satisfy them, when it comes to what is at stake for them – their secrets, their secret *jouissance* – they want to hold on to it. In obsession we find essentially a desire to retain, in that sense it is an anal desire, the desire to retain the object from the Other, the object the Other is supposed to want (Silvestre 2018, 97). This makes the task of the analyst difficult. When the obsessional is confronted with the desire of the Other which requires that he must give up something, he may leave. But this confrontation has to happen at some point in the analysis.

What insists for the obsessional is the pull to return to the lost *jouissance* which at the same time gives rise to anxiety and which the obsessional does not want to know anything about (Silvestre 2018, 99). Hence, the treatment should address the subject's position in relation to *jouissance*, rather than aim primarily at revealing repressed material (Voruz and Wolf 2007, xiv). It should be directed at the lack and the object that stands in place of the lack that evokes *jouissance* and that the obsessional doesn't want to let go of. In the analytic process the analysand "has the chance to encounter and confront his lack, rather than avoid it, and to assume the desire arising from it. This entails a process of separation", separation from the object and the *jouissance* it promises, that leads to greater freedom than the obsessional manoeuvres to keep the Other at a distance (Gessert 2014, 66–67).

This can become possible if the analyst positions himself "in the very place where the event has triggered something overwhelming for the subject" (Silvestre

2018, 103). We can see this with the Rat Man when he became very agitated, confusing Freud with the captain and with his father who used to beat him. The analyst must bring desire for knowledge to bear, as when Freud asked for the photo of the lady; he must insist that there is more to know than what is obvious, that there is not one fixed meaning, that there is something beyond the meanings the patient, and perhaps the analyst, provide, that it is the knowledge about *jouissance* that constitutes the patient's truth (Silvestre 2018, 109).

But this is not what the patient is looking for and it is not where he positions the analyst in the transference. In the transference the typical obsessional's relation to the Other will appear; they will be either the "perfect" patient, scrupulously providing what they think the analyst demands, like the Rat Man who produced a wealth of material, or they will be distant, monosyllabic in their responses, "rejecting anything that comes from the Other". Either way, they destroy the potential for any fundamental shift to occur in their relation to the Other, to desire, and *jouissance* (Verhaeghe 2018, 394). They may try to take over the treatment process and the analyst, literally talking over him, providing their own interpretations, rejecting any ideas that do not fit into their system – as the Rat Man did with Freud's interpretations about his hostile feelings towards his father – and they do this in a typical obsessional way, demonstrating their own mastery and independence.

In such cases, patients may leave prematurely, they find the analyst is no match for them, they think they know much more and are much more sophisticated (Verhaeghe 2018, 394–395). If they stay, they may position the analyst as master who knows something about how to regulate the *jouissance* of which they do not want to know anything. They want the analyst to take care of it so that they can carry on as before in their own sweet ways (Silvestre 2018, 109, 113). This can be a strong temptation for the analyst, to take up a position of mastery, to provide meanings and make interpretations in the form of injunctions that will banish desire, *jouissance*, and lack from the treatment (p. 109). This will help "to block out … anxiety, but the price … will be a reinforcement of his neurosis" and the analysis becomes interminable (pp. 95, 113). Freud did take up the position of master to some extent, when he said to the Rat Man that he would guess what he wanted to say; when the patient could not speak, Freud provided words for him; and he gave him a meal when he was hungry. In these instances, rather than allowing for lack and desire to arise, Freud closed the gap (see Mahony 2007).

This is also the problem with interpretations through which meaning is produced. The meaning of the symptom may become clear, and the symptom may disappear. For instance, the Rat Man's *jouissance* had become symbolised in his procrastinations, in his failure to complete his studies, which Freud interpreted as manifestations of his conflict about marrying the lady. But later in life, after the analysis, the symptom returned, the Rat Man showed instability in his professional career, moving from office to office (Mahony 2007, 109).

Providing meaning does not touch on the drive that is enveloped in the symptom and keeps circulating around the object. It is this real of the symptom, the kernel of *jouissance* that is related to the drive that resists conventional analytic work through interpretation that aims at the dissolution of the symptom by lifting the repression and providing meaning. Even when repression is lifted, when the unconscious has been made conscious by finding words for it – which is the usual aim of traditional analysis – the drive root of the symptom remains still intact. When the signifying structures of the subject's identifications have been dismantled, the drive has still remained untouched and can insert itself again into another chain of signifiers (see Verhaeghe and Declercq 2016, 337–338, 346). It is this real root of the symptom where the *jouissance* is located that the obsessional has to acknowledge and confront. In his later teaching period, Lacan emphasised the dual function of language. Language is not only a means of reducing *jouissance*, of regulating the drive, it is also a means of enjoyment (Voruz & Wolf 2007, ix). Obsessionals especially can indulge in this type of enjoyment, constructing complex systems of thought – what the Rat Man called *Gedankenarbeit* (thought work) – with many false connections, ellipses, loose ends, and isolated phrases. It is this same enjoyment that they need to surrender (Solano-Suàrez 2007, 97–98).

To expose the real kernel of the symptom, the symbolic wrapping of the symptom has to be dismantled to reveal the void behind the object that stands for the lacking thing, and the *jouissance* related to it. Interpretation, in the classic sense of pointing to another meaning and lifting the repression, is not sufficient to achieve this aim. It introduces more signifying material, it encourages meaning-making and the enjoyment that comes with it. What must finally become revealed through the process of analysis is not meaning, but the non-sense of the symptoms the analysand presents, the enjoyment involved in them, and the lack that is covered by them. The subject must acknowledge this enjoyment and not hold on to it, but in a sense take hold of it. When this happens, the analysand can put something else, another, *better* symptom in this void (Verhaeghe and Declercq 2016, 337–338, 345; Lacan [1964] 1994, 250–251; 1974–1975, 106–107). For this to happen, the analysis will still address the symbolic constructions of the analysand, but the analyst should also aim at opening a space for lack to disrupt the situation of immobility and to confront the patient with the enigma of his lack and his desire (see Verhaeghe and Declercq 2016, 341).

There are many ways of doing this. Working with variable session times can be one way of creating a lack, of keeping something in suspense. But there are also other interventions that confront the analysand with an enigma rather than with meaning, such as changing the punctuation of the analysand's speech, picking up an apparently irrelevant detail, using equivocations, asking analysands to complete their sentences where they broke them off, marking unprovoked denials. Such interventions indicate that there is more to know, that something remains unrecognised (Solano-Suàrez 2007, 99).

For such work to become possible, both analysand and analyst have to give up their belief in the Other as an all-powerful father, as final guarantee that there is an ultimate meaning, an ultimate truth, an ultimate object that can solve the dilemma of the human subject. Freud had taken the position of this Other as powerful father in the transference. By his own account, taking too much the position of the father disqualified him "as a great analyst" (Kardiner 1977, 69; Verhaeghe and Declercq 2016, 352). He had placed the father in the place of the lack of the Other. Rather than believing that there is an object that can make him or the Other complete, the analysand can realise through the analysis that he and the Other will always lack something, that the Other does not have the answer, he does not have what would complete him, and that his identities are always "an alienation in the signifiers of the Other" (Verhaeghe and Declercq 2016, 351–352; see also Verhaeghe 1998, 100, 103–104). On reaching this point, the subject can build his identity not only out of signifiers that come from an Other, but he can also define himself through his own particular way of enjoying. He supplements for the lack, not by creating symptoms with the use of signifiers given by others, but by using his own drive and enjoyment to create a new symptom, independent of the Other. This, we might say, is a *real* separation from this Other.

We might wonder if in our world today such a realisation is more difficult to achieve than in Freud's time with its many restrictions. Today's mentality might support the illusion that the ultimate object of satisfaction does actually exist, and not only this, but that it can also be reached for really or virtually, that it can be bought, that we can have the ultimate experience that is so often advertised and promised (Verhaeghe 2018, 170, note 20).

References

Freud, Sigmund. (1907–1908). "Addendum: Original Record of the Case". In *The Standard Edition of the Complete Psychological Works of Sigmund Freud*, translated by James Strachey, vol. 10, pp. 259–318. London: Hogarth, 1955.

Freud, Sigmund. (1909). "Notes Upon a Case of Obsessional Neurosis". In *The Standard Edition of the Complete Psychological Works of Sigmund Freud*, translated by James Strachey, vol. 10, pp. 151–249. London: Hogarth, 1955.

Freud, Sigmund. (1926). "Inhibitions, Symptoms, and Anxiety". In *The Standard Edition of the Complete Psychological Works of Sigmund Freud*, translated by James Strachey, vol. 20, pp. 75–175. London: Hogarth, 1959.

Gessert, Astrid. (2014). "Hysteria and Obsession". In *Introductory Lectures on Lacan*, edited by Astrid Gessert, pp. 55–68. London: Karnac.

Kardiner, Abram. (1977). *My Analysis with Freud: Reminiscences*. New York: Norton.

Lacan, Jacques. (1959–1960). *The Ethics of Psychoanalysis*. In *The Seminar of Jacques Lacan, Book VII*, translated by Denis Porter, edited by Jacques-Alain Miller. New York: Norton, 1992.

Lacan, Jacques. (1964). *The Four Fundamental Concepts of Psychoanalysis*. In *The Seminar of Jacques Lacan, Book XI*, translated by Alan Sheridan, edited by Jacques-Alain Miller. London: Penguin, 1994.

Lacan, Jacques. (1974–1975). R.S.I. *Ornicar? Bulletin périodique du champ Freudien [Journal of the Freudian Field]*, 3.

Mahony, Patrick. (2007). "Reading the Notes on the Rat Man Case: Freud's Own Obsessional Character and Mother Complex". *Canadian Journal of Psychoanalysis* 15(1): 93–117.

Melman, Charles. (2018). "The Rat Man". In *Obsessional Neurosis: Lacanian Perspectives*, edited by Astrid Gessert, pp. 83–92. Abingdon: Routledge.

Silvestre, Michel. (2018). "The Lacanian Structure of Obsessional Neurosis". In *Obsessional Neurosis: Lacanian Perspectives*, edited by Astrid Gessert, pp. 93–120. Abingdon: Routledge.

Solano-Suàrez, Esthela. (2007). "Identification with the Symptom at the End of Analysis". In *The Later Lacan*, edited by Veronique Voruz and Bogdan Wolf, pp. 95–104. Albany, NY: State University of New York Press.

Vanheule, Stijn. (2001). "Inhibition: 'I Am Because I Don't Act'". *The Letter* 23, 109–126.

Verhaeghe, Paul. (1998). "Trauma and Hysteria in Freud and Lacan". *The Letter* 14, 87–105.

Verhaeghe, Paul. (2018). *On Being Normal and Other Disorders*. Abingdon: Routledge.

Verhaeghe, Paul and Declercq, Frederic. (2016). "Lacan's Analytic Goal: Le Sinthome or the Feminine Way". *Psychoanalytische Perspectieven* 34(4), 336–357.

Voruz, Veronique and Wolf, Bogdan. (2007). "Preface". In *The Later Lacan*, edited by Veronique Voruz and Bogdan Wolf, pp. vii–xvii. Albany, NY: State University of New York Press.

Chapter 8

Freud's Knight

Guy Le Gaufey

Freud's 1909 text "*Bemerkungen über einen Fall von Zwangsneurose*" ["Notes Upon a Case of Obsessional Neurosis"] must be read today as an historical document. It is no longer a text we can naively read with the idea that we are or want to be Freudian and are in a direct connection with it. This is not only because time has passed and the general culture has changed, but because the stakes that were Freud's at the time cannot be precisely ours today. If obsessional neurosis still exists nowadays – no doubt about it – the Rat Man case is no longer the model we can trust as a timeless standard. Furthermore, the psychoanalytic classification of hysteria, obsession, phobia, perversion, and psychosis is as useful today as Esquirol's monomania or Bleuler's schizophrenia. I do not think that we have better naming today and I do not trust the DSM-IV or the DSM-V more. I suspect that *structures* and the theoretical field they refer to are nothing but a first step for the psychoanalytic clinical field, a step that deserves to be surpassed if we want to consider… transference. As long as the analyst is a *clinician*, s/he is bound to refer to structures and nosographic categories (Le Gaufey 2007) and in remaining in that clinical stance throughout the treatment, transference will be out of reach or it will turn into another piece of clinical knowledge which leaves the analyst out of the process and conscious only of what s/he calls "countertransference", a term that assumes that the analyst is merely answering the patient's transference. I will try to make clear that Freud's own transference with the Rat Man is not just a mode of reply to his patient but is undoubtedly the starting point of the case.

To establish such a point, I will refer to four different texts. First, there is Freud's "Notes Upon a Case of Obsessional Neurosis" (Freud 1909) but equally the famous "Journal" which was published partially and then later in English under the title "Addendum: Original Record of the Case" in a Strachey translation (Freud 1907–1908). I will refer to the complete French and bilingual publication by Elza Ribeiro Hawelka in 1974. Moreover, I will use two other texts which I recommend if you want to know more about the Rat Man and diversify points of view on the case. The first is the text that gives us all of the information about the case itself and the true civil name of the Rat Man, Ernst Lanzer, as well as the family history and historical details including some that were unavailable to Freud at the time of the treatment. This is a precious book published by Patrick Mahony in 1986 called *Freud and the*

DOI: 10.4324/9781032663746-13

Ratman. Finally, there is Lacan's "The Neurotic's Individual Myth", which is a talk given in Paris in 1952 at the Collège Philosophique. Thanks to these very different and coherent readings, we will be in a position to *return to Freud* because we will be able to assess how far from us Freud is now regarding his technique, and how close to us he is regarding transference. As Freud himself says in the middle of his twenty-seventh lecture on "Transference", and after speaking for pages and pages without mentioning even once the word "transference", he says, in a very theatrical style, "*Und nun, die Tatsache*" [And now for the facts] (Freud 1917 [1916–1917], 437). Let's do the same now.

On 1 October 1907 – it was then a Tuesday afternoon – the aforementioned Ernst Lanzer comes into Freud's office for the first time. I can only guess that within minutes Freud already knew that before him was what was later named in American analysts' offices during the 1960s and 1970s a *YAVIS* syndrome. I have been told that this acronym has all but disappeared, but it seems to me very appropriate as a description of this first encounter. YAVIS means "young, attractive, verbally fluent, intelligent and sophisticated". Ernst Lanzer was all that to Freud who had been waiting for this kind of patient for a rather long time. We are going to learn for how long exactly.

In order not to rush into the Rat Man case as the paradigm it has become for a century, it is worth considering in what circumstances it took place for Freud. At the beginning of 1896, Freud, who wrote at least weekly to his friend Wilhelm Fliess, sent him what he called "Manuscript K" that dealt with "The Neuroses of Defence", with a humoristic subtitle, "A Christmas Fairy Tale" (Freud 1896a, 220–229). He revealed here in detail his fiery ideas about obsessional neurosis, hysteria, and paranoia. He then wrote, "The course of events in obsessional neurosis is what is clearest to me, because I have come to know it best" (Masson 1985, 164).

There are many reasons for such a belief. Contrary to the main idea that Freud began mostly with hysteria because of "Studies on Hysteria", he was more interested in the treatment of obsession. His colleagues of that time recognised that they failed to cure patients of their obsessions and anxiety, whereas with hysteria they could think of themselves as being as successful as Freud while using different modes of therapy. A therapeutic success with obsessional neurosis would have functioned as a proof of the correctness of Freud's general theory regarding psychic organisation. The key point, already present in his text, "Further Remarks on the Neuro-Psychoses of Defence" (Freud 1896b), is the separation between affect and idea – representation or *Vorstellung*. In the second part of this text, "Nature and Mechanism of Obsessional Neurosis," Freud unveils the nature of obsessional neurosis as follows: "The nature of obsessional neurosis can be expressed in a simple formula. *Obsessional ideas* are invariably transformed *self-reproaches* which have re-emerged from *repression* and which always relate to some *sexual* act that was performed with pleasure in *childhood*" (Freud 1896b, 169, italics in original).

Because repression has separated affect from idea regarding the active and pleasant sexual act in early childhood, contrary to hysteria where the seduction is supposed to have been passive, the repressed idea will reappear consciously most of the time as something absurd – because it is disconnected from its original affect – while the original affect itself will appear as shame, or hypochondriac anxiety, or social or religious angst, or even observation mania, all of which are a group of *obsessional affects*. What was central in the explanation of obsessional ideas for Freud's colleagues working in this therapeutic field, including Breuer and many others, is moral consciousness. This moral consciousness was no longer at stake for Freud in his new understanding of the *psychic mechanism* which produces obsessional states.

Into this Viennese battlefield of the mid-1890s came the case of Mr. E. who appeared in Freud's correspondence with Wilhelm Fliess. Mr. E. first appeared in a letter on 4 November 1895 and repeatedly over five years which was a long treatment according to Freud's standards in this matter at that time. We get some information from time to time about him in these correspondences. In a letter dated 21 December 1899, which was close to the end of the treatment, Freud eventually gave Fliess a lengthy explanation:

> You are familiar with my dream which obstinately promises the end of E's treatment (among the absurd dreams), and you can well imagine how important this one persistent patient has become to me. It now appears that the dream will be fulfilled. I cautiously say "appears," but I am really quite certain. Buried deep beneath all his fantasies, we found a scene from his primal period (before twenty-two months) which meets all the requirements and in which all the remaining puzzles converge. It is everything at the same time—sexual, innocent, natural, and the rest. I scarcely dare believe it yet. It is as if Schliemann had once more excavated Troy, which had hitherto been deemed a fable. At the same time the fellow is doing outrageously well. He demonstrated the reality of my theory in my own case, providing me a surprising reversal with the solution, which I had overlooked, to my former railroad phobia. For this piece of work, I even made him the present of a picture of Œdipus and the Sphinx.
>
> (Masson 1985, 391–392)

Six months later and after five years of treatment, there eventually came the last day of E.'s treatment on April 16, 1900, and Freud wrote:

> E. at last concluded his career as a patient by coming to dinner at my house. His riddle is almost completely solved, he is in excellent shape, his personality entirely changed. At present, a remnant of the symptoms is left. I am beginning to understand that the apparent endlessness of the treatment is something that occurs regularly and is connected with transference … In any case, I shall keep an eye on the man. Since he had to suffer through all my technical and theoretical errors, I actually think that a future case could be solved in half the time. May the Lord now send this next one.
>
> (Masson 1985, 409)[1]

Seven and a half years later, both this last wish and humoristic entreaty were fulfilled when on 1 October 1907, Ernst Lanzer made his entrance into Freud's office. We know that Freud had great expectations regarding his own need to perfect his conception of obsessional neurosis. Fliess had by then disappeared as the *publicum* he had been for ten years but from 1902 the Wednesday Society – a group of those whom Freud later called with a certain disdain "my Viennese" – used to meet with him every Wednesday. From 1906, these meetings sometimes included visitors who were passing through such as Jung, Abraham, or Ferenczi. This group was the addressee of the construction Freud built from the very first of Lanzer's sessions. I will mention only two facts that are very revealing about Freud's attitude to this most welcome case.

At the Wednesday meeting of 6 November 1907, less than one month after the first encounter and after only a few sessions, Freud spoke of the patient already named "the Rat Man" to his Viennese audience (Nunberg 1976, 246)). Let's not forget that the Wednesday meetings took place until 1910 in Freud's apartment and that as a rule, it was required that every participant spoke at least a few words. Silence was prohibited. Captain Freud was adamant on this point.

Moreover, during the Salzburg Congress on 27 April 1908, while the Rat Man was still on the couch – his analysis lasted for 11 months, according to Freud – Freud spoke for four hours without a break about the Rat Man in front of 42 people. When he stopped, the audience, which included Jung, Abraham, Ferenczi, and Jones, urged him to go further. He agreed and continued for another hour (Jones 1961, 44). Five hours were thus solely dedicated to the Rat Man – between two sessions with him, of course. In addition, Freud had spoken on four occasions about the Rat Man at the Wednesday meetings: on 20 November 22 January, 4 March and 8 April and each time he added new pieces to the case. He was clearly ready for his performance at the end of April in Salzburg.

Why was there such conspicuousness from the very beginning to the final writing of the case? The first pages of the case are very clear on that topic:

> It was a complete obsessional neurosis, wanting in no essential element, at once the nucleus and the prototype of the later disorder—an elementary organism, as it were, the study of which could alone enable us to obtain a grasp of the complicated organization of his subsequent illness.
>
> (Freud 1909, 162)

And what are we supposed to find out in this "prototype"? A few lines later, Freud explains this when he enumerates three different couples of antagonistic terms:

> We find, accordingly: an erotic instinct and a revolt against it; a wish which has not yet become compulsive and, struggling against it, a fear which is already compulsive; a distressing affect and an impulsion towards the performance of defensive acts. The inventory of the neurosis has reached its full muster [*das Inventar der Neurose ist vollzählig*].
>
> (Freud 1909, 163)

This is really the marvel Freud had waited for since 16 April 1900. Should we ourselves still be trapped by such a persuasive rhetoric? That is the point we must shed some light on. If we want to be positively critical, we first need to properly establish why Freud is so satisfied by the case itself.

I will not meander into the many labyrinthine aspects of the case because to make them comprehensible would take too long and submit us to a non-critical attitude because we would spend all of our time quoting Freud's text or, worse, summing it up. One indispensable approach is a close reading – or a *re-reading* – of the case and, if possible, a linked reading of the "Journal" or the less complete English version "Record of the Case" (Freud 1907–1908). Both are good pieces of literature. The "Journal" is the daily report of the first sessions, and it is enthralling.

I would prefer to stress something that is trickier to perceive through the many events, names, thoughts, and other considerations, theoretical and practical. According to the previous quotation, the nucleus of obsessional neurosis is composed of strong oppositions between terms that are constitutively conflictual: an instinct – according to Strachey, but in fact, *eine erotischer Trieb* (an erotic drive) – and a revolt (*Auflehnung*) against it; a wish (*ein Wunsch*) and a fear (*eine Befürchtung*); a distressing affect and an "impulsion" – in fact, *ein Drang*, a term belonging already to the vocabulary of drive "pressure" – towards defence.

But what kind of conflict is at stake in those pairings? On the one hand, a first indication comes from a lexicographic reading. The word *ambivalence* is mentioned only once, in a note and in reference to Bleuler (Freud 1909, 239, fn, 1). Freud does not use this term which is so frequently used in the Freudian world for lazy explanations about too many things. On the other hand, the word *conflict* is used here in the Rat Man case 26 times and *struggle* 12 times. This is approximately 36 occurrences of a conflict through which the psychic apparatus is structured. Thus, in the same way hysteria functioned as a proof of the existence of deferred action and the decisive play of fantasy, obsessional neurosis could be perceived as pursued by Freud as proof of the conflictual nature of psychic life that he is so attached to.

Is *conflict* so central a notion in psychoanalysis? For now, I worry about the importance we are supposed to give to it because of Freud's insistence. It is obvious that there are local conflicts between different elements, different agencies, different wishes, and anywhere in psychic life a conflict can emerge. But is it truly fundamental? Such a question is enough to begin to foresee something which is in fact so frequent, so natural, so obvious throughout Freud's texts that we do not pay enough attention to it: his deep dualism.

I do not forget that the first and second topologies are composed of three terms – Ucs/Pcs/Cs (ego, id, superego) but the relationships between their different elements are exclusively dualistic and conflictual, especially in the second topology. And I do not forget a little fact: Freud was invited in May 1910 by the great and famous physicist Wilhelm Ostwald (the 1909 Nobel Prize winner, no less) to write a paper that would be published in the *Annalen der Naturphilosophie*, a journal openly in favour of energeticism. This energeticism was in fact a monism which considered that at the bottom of the physical world only energy exists. Freud, honoured by the invitation, wrote to Jung saying that after reflection he would say "yes", only to then discard it and not write anything, refusing to take psychoanalysis in the direction of monism, and returning to his natural dualism. This dualism was to prevail in "Beyond the Pleasure Principle" (Freud 1920) with the life drive and death drive.

To shed more light on this point, I will refer briefly to a discovery made by the American historian of sciences, Gerald Holton. He observed that frequently a central idea in the building of a scientific theory will be omitted in the final index. Why? Because this idea occurs throughout the text as something so obvious, so natural, so inescapable that it is beyond any kind of definition or experimentation. For instance, what is behind the apparent complexity of phenomena, and what is primal in physical reality; is it order or disorder? In classical physics, for Kepler, Galileo and Newton, order was primal and thanks to Kepler's laws, it was possible to approach, behind the apparent disorder of the movements of the planets, a perfect regularity of the real world. At base, ontologically, not epistemologically, was order. By contrast, around 1850 when thermodynamics was central to physics, it was thought the ultimate reality behind the apparent calm of gas in a bottle was the ceaseless Brownian movement of molecules. At the basis was disorder. Then, in 1905, Einstein demonstrated that this movement of molecules could be described in a classical way and once again, at the basis was order (Holton 1978, 3–24).

It is the same with quantum physics. Is the statistical disorder of particles the true and ultimate truth? Werner Heisenberg and Niels Bohr thought so. Einstein, however, forced to recognise the experimental validity and success of this quantum physics, thought that later with new technical means "variables that are still hidden" will be discovered and will prove that what is behind all that mess is nothing but order and regularity – "The Lord does not play dice." Holton proposed to name these basic convictions "themata" with this subsequent definition, "a prototype of explanation that is a thematic commitment. It is not an experimental or a logical necessity" (Holton 1978, 20).

Freud's dualism, as such, is to be considered as a themata and, in this perspective, the Rat Man as his knight. He ceaselessly clashes with any and all ideas, struggles against any and all affects, combats any and all transferences. With him, everything is potentially a fight, and all of that was exhausting, so it is no surprise that on 1 October 1907, in front of Freud, Ernst Lanzer is worn-out.

Is this a reason to be dubious about Freud's conception of obsessional neurosis or about Freudian psychoanalysis in general? No, I do not think so. By stressing Freud's dualism as a themata, I want to introduce the idea that when the word *nature* is used as an argument – and let us recall that Freud said, "the *nature* of obsessional neurosis can be expressed ..." (as above, Freud 1896, 169) – something which is not so *natural* was previously and necessarily introduced. This is a *themata commitment*. We must be attentive to what this achieves, this silent and omnipresent commitment without which the writer would have been incapable of constructing and construing anything.

I am therefore in favour of a comparative approach to the case which allows me to turn to Lacan, since I am in the position of an old Lacanian. "Le mythe individual du névrosé" ["The Neurotic's Individual Myth"] was a talk given by Lacan in 1952 and includes a commentary on Freud's Rat Man text, followed by one on Goethe's *Poetry and Truth*. In his seminars, Lacan did speak from time to time about the Rat Man, but it was mostly a reiteration of what he said in this talk which came just before he began his teaching.

Once again, I offer a lexicographic remark: if you peruse Lacan's text about the case itself, you will encounter only three mentions of the word *conflit* [conflict]. The last mention, which is of no value to us, is "assumer les fruits de son travail *sans conflit*" (Lacan [1952] 2007, 32) ["to accept the fruits of his work without conflict"].[2] This poses no problem. The concept of *conflit* is not at work here. Then there is "le conflit femme riche/femme pauvre" (p. 23) ["the conflict between the rich and the poor woman"].[3] This is only a reminder to us of Freud's own expression, and Lacan is stressing the repetition from the father to his son Ernst regarding whom he is to be married to. In the third and final occurrence, Lacan writes "une espèce de conflit anxieux, si caractéristique du vécu des obsessionnels" (p. 26) [one of these conflicts is so characteristic of obsessionals' experience"].[4] I'll leave it to you to appreciate the fact that in this sentence the key word is not *conflict* but the idea of *scenario*.

In fact, this quasi absence of the notion of conflict in Lacan's text is not surprising. The next year after making these remarks, he launched in 1953 his "thériaque" (an ancient medicine made of many different elements belonging to *three* different orders: mineral, vegetal, and animal), meaning his three basic concepts of symbolic, imaginary and real, which were to escort him up to the Borromean knots and his last seminars. Similar to Charles Sanders Peirce, Lacan is someone who begins by counting three, at first. As in the Christian Trinity, the unity comes after having put together a primal and immediate triplicity into which each term is as powerful as the two others. I won't go further into this matter of theoretical consistency in Lacan's teaching, but I introduce this perspective to understand why his commentary about the Rat Man follows scrupulously some pieces of the narration of events given by Freud, and yet develops such a different sense of it. This is not really a matter of analytical concepts as at this time Lacan had not formulated his special concept of *subject*, nor *object a*, and even the notion of *signifier* is far from being clear. This latter will only appear for the first time at the end of December 1961, at the beginning of the seminar on *Identification*. It is a question of basic themata and Lacan is in no way following a dualistic pattern or in a conflictual universe, so his clinical perspective is subtly and constantly different from Freud's. That means that an event or transference is understood and described by Lacan as an articulated sequence – a *scenario* as in "The Purloined Letter" (Lacan [1955] 2006) – whereas Freud stresses an antagonistic opposition as soon as it is rationally available.

The funny thing is that, in this text, and even more in his commentary on Goethe, Lacan is in favour of a symbolic *quatuor* (a quartet). He does so after having announced that "the whole schema of Œdipus is to be criticised" (Lacan [1952]

2007, 44), proposing the introduction of a fourth element in the Œdipus triangulation: death. But he never proposed any kind of dualism, and his Rat Man is a sort of champion of the symbolic order, with his debt as impossible to cancel as was the one his father had failed to pay back: this is pure repetition in the symbolic chain. The point which Lacan insists on most often is the moment when the Rat Man opens the door at night to his dead father before he (the Rat Man) masturbates. This obsession is precious to Lacan because he is then trying to establish his own concept of "symbolic phallus", "big phi", an interpretation you would search in vain for in Freud, but which has a valuable role in considering the big Other's desire in obsessional ideas and repetitive acts.

Where am I going with these remarks? I am trying to make clear that the word *clinic*, as paramount as it is in our practice, deserves to be considered cautiously. I am struck, for instance, by the success recently encountered by the expression, "In my clinic, I…" in English as in French. I do not understand this possessive adjective. I can say *my practice* because it is something private, but *clinic* cannot be *mine* so easily. It is what I try to partially establish when I work with colleagues, with texts I read or write. It is a construction that I build from my practice with patients, my *thematas*, my own neurosis, and some other ingredients. It is never something *natural*.

The Rat Man is perfect for this kind of exercise: to build a little piece of clinic from the different texts at our disposal, from our clinical experience, our theoretical preferences, our present convictions about what psychoanalysis must be, and so on. You notice that I said "our". I mean that it is difficult to conceive of *clinic* as a solitary work. In my opinion, one of the most decisive inventions Lacan made when he founded the *École Freudienne de Paris* was the *cartel*. More than three and less than seven people – more than the Graces, less than the Muses – gathered for a while in an uncertain chemistry, without hierarchy, speaking freely around a commonly chosen theme. That is for me the true laboratory from which elements of the clinic can emerge.

That is why I will turn now to Mahony's book. It is precious, especially to English readers, because he introduces some critical commentaries about Strachey's translation, using the German text. These commentaries allow us to take some distance from the English text. They allow us to conceive that an idea was primarily put in another way, with another semantic context, often this is the first step in freeing the signified from the signifiers. For instance, in Freud's narrations (of dreams, of scenes, of obsessional ideas), Strachey systematically puts the verbs in the past tense, whereas Freud keeps the present time, and the enunciation is therefore quite different. Where Freud writes *our* patient, Strachey puts *the* patient. These slight differences eventually are very important when you care about the analyst's transference, which is precisely what we should do.

But Mahony offers us more in including a detailed explanation about why Freud was so dissatisfied with this text. He was clearly overwhelmed by the abundance of data that Ernst Lanzer threw at him ceaselessly. This is indicated in his passing from "*Remarks*" to "*Notes*" and even to "*Aphorisms* about a Case of

Obsessional Neurosis". thus admitting to not being able to frame it. He felt forced to let the different threads go their way, with each conflict deserving its own description, with no possibility of reducing all of it to a single psychical mechanism. That is also why Freud's text is so difficult to grasp, so open to different types of commentaries and theoretical perspectives. Although the Rat Man has been presented from the very beginning as a *nucleus*, a *prototype*, a sort of paradigm, the text itself keeps offering an abundance of divergent data to each reader. This abundance partly explains why Freud was so talkative each time he spoke about the case. It also explains why Freud's text is at the same time stunning and disappointing – this last term being far from being negative in my mind. I do agree with Mahony's final words regarding Freud's style as "magnificence in failure" (Mahony 1986, 243).

I will conclude with this term *failure*. This is not to magnify the failure itself but to find in it the mark of true humanity. No, that sounds too Christian to me. I just want to shed some light on the analytical treatment of obsessional neurosis. It is well known that these kinds of treatment are reputed to be interminable and therefore especially boring. On this point, let me tell you a story concerning Wilfred Bion. It seems he received for a long time a man he considered to be a serious obsessional. This patient was apparently so boring that during each afternoon session Bion was very close to falling asleep. One day, he asked himself "But how does he manage to bore me so much?" and out of the blue, with this single question, this patient became very interesting. The boredom was momentarily suspended, and the treatment proceeded differently. Unfortunately, I don't know how it all turned out, but thanks to this kind of story we can appreciate Lacan's assertion that the analyst is half of the patient's symptom when this symptom has taken on its transferential value.

Let us now return to Freud's failure, according to Mahony. If it is to be understood as a mark of incompleteness, pointing to the fact that Freud repetitively struggled to *close* his narration, we must therefore consider this point as decisive regarding the consistency of the clinic we are trying to learn about and construct. With the term *closing*, I mean a conclusion that would bring together the main threads of the narration, offering the reader a capacity of memorisation that comes from a feeling of unity. With this, the various data scattered throughout the text supposedly converge in an imaginary form, very often hanging on only a very few words, thus providing a unity of meaning generally considered as a definition. This is something we first aim at in a clinical elaboration: to get a *picture* of the *case*. But if we stop at such a point, we seriously miss our position of analyst and become forgetful of transference.

In reading not the *case* but the *writing of the case*, we can see how Freud is constantly torn between his aspirations towards the definitive *nucleus* he promises, and the intricate net of events, remembrances, transferences, obsessional ideas that the *Journal/Record* is full of. This split in Freud's research is our chance not to be trapped in a purely imaginary approach to *THE* obsessional as has happened throughout history, culture, and analytical schools.

Notes

1 In German, it is *Der Herr send nun diesen nächsten* (Masson 1985, 449).
2 My translation.
3 My translation.
4 My translation.

References

Freud, Sigmund. (1896a). "*Draft K: The Neuroses of Defence (A Christmas Fairy Tale)*". In *The Standard Edition of the Complete Psychological Works of Sigmund Freud*, edited by James Strachey, vol. 1, pp. 220–229. London: Hogarth. 1955.

Freud, Sigmund. (1896b). "Further Remarks on the Neuro-Psychoses of Defence". In *The Standard Edition of the Complete Psychological Works of Sigmund Freud*, edited by James Strachey, vol. 3, pp. 157–185. London: Hogarth, 1955.

Freud, Sigmund. (1907–1908). "Addendum: Original Record of the Case". In *The Standard Edition of the Complete Psychological Works of Sigmund Freud*, edited by James Strachey, vol. 10, pp. 259–318. London: Hogarth, 1955.

Freud, Sigmund. (1909). "Notes Upon a Case of Obsessional Neurosis". In *The Standard Edition of the Complete Psychological Works of Sigmund Freud*, edited by James Strachey, vol. 10, pp. 155–249. London: Hogarth, 1955.

Freud, Sigmund. (1917 [1916–1917]). "Lecture XXVII: Transference". In *The Standard Edition of the Complete Psychological Works of Sigmund Freud*, edited by James Strachey, vol. 16, pp. 431–447. London: Hogarth, 1955.

Freud, Sigmund. (1920). "Beyond the Pleasure Principle". In *The Standard Edition of the Complete Psychological Works of Sigmund Freud*, edited by James Strachey, vol. 18, pp. 7–64. London: Hogarth. 1955.

Hawalka, Elza Ribeiro. (1974). *L'Homme aux rats: Journal d'une analyse par Sigmund Freud*. Paris: Presses Universitaires de France.

Holton, Gerald. (1978). *The Scientific Imagination*. Cambridge: Cambridge University Press.

Jones, Ernest. (1961). *La Vie et l'œuvre de Sigmund Freud*, vol. II. Paris: PUF.

Lacan, Jacques. (1952). *Le Mythe individuel du névrosé*. Paris: Seuil, 2007.

Lacan, Jacques. (1955). Seminar on "The Purloined Letter". In *Écrits: The First Complete Edition in English*, translated by Bruce Fink, pp. 4–48. New York: Norton, 2006.

Le Gaufey, Guy. (2007). "Is the Analyst a Clinician?" *Journal for the Centre for Freudian Analysis and Research, JCFAR*, 17.

Mahony, Patrick. (1986). *Freud and the Ratman*. New Haven, CT: Yale University Press.

Masson, Jeffrey. M. (ed.) (1985). *The Complete Letters of Sigmund Freud to Wilhelm Fliess (1987–1904)*. London: Belknap Press.

Nunberg, Herman. (1976). *Les Premiers Psychanalystes. Minutes de la Société psychanalytique de Vienne, 1906–1908*, vol. I. Paris: Gallimard.

THE WOLF MAN

From the History of an Infantile Neurosis

SERGIUS (SERGEI) KONSTANTINOVICH PANKEJEFF

Born 24 December 1886, near Kherson, Ukraine
Died 7 May 1979, Steinhof Psychiatric Hospital, Vienna

This-is-what-must-have-happened

Freud, Sigmund. (1918). "From the History of an
Infantile Neurosis". In *The Standard Edition of the
Complete Psychological Works of Sigmund Freud*, translated by
James Strachey, vol. 17, pp. 7–122. London: Hogarth, 1955.

DOI: 10.4324/9781032663746-14

Chapter 9

The Wolf Man, Invented

Annie G. Rogers

The Original Invention

Let us begin with the original invention by Freud, who gave Sergei Pankejeff the name Wolf Man – naming him for a signature dream about wolves – and the diagnosis of obsessional.

Let us also begin by considering how Sergei ended up with Freud and what happened. In January 1910, Sergei Pankejeff's physician brought him to Vienna for treatment in a sanitorium. Pankejeff, who had been treated for gonorrhoea and had already been diagnosed as manic depressive, now presented with an inability to have a bowel movement without an enema, as well as continuing debilitating depression which interrupted all his normal life activities and interests. After a short stay at a sanitorium, Pankejeff chose to begin a psychoanalytic treatment with Freud. They met each other between February 1910 and July 1914, a long analysis at the time. Freud saw Pankejeff again several times beyond the end of this first analysis, including a brief second analysis in 1919. For several years, according to Freud, Pankejeff resisted the analysis. He did so by accepting interpretations passively, with no result whatsoever, until Freud gave him a one-year deadline for the termination of the analysis, prompting Pankejeff to *give up his resistances* (Freud 1918b, 209). Freud's first publication of the "Wolf Man" was "From the History of an Infantile Neurosis" (*Aus der Geschichte einer infantilen Neurose*), written at the end of 1914 but not published until 1918. I am using Aday Huish's (Freud 1918b) relatively recent and very good translation of Freud's case in preference to the text of the Standard Edition. I chose this because the Standard Edition has not only been standardised but also medicalised and a good translation of Freud's German does not have this problem.

A Light Sketch of Childhood History

As a child, Sergei was initially a calm, quiet character. As a result of this and his sister's boisterous behaviour, he recalled having been told by his parents that he should have born a girl and she a boy. However, the boy's parents found a dramatic change in his attitude when they returned from holiday on one occasion. The boy had become argumentative, irritable, and sometimes violent. His parents suspected

DOI: 10.4324/9781032663746-15

that this was a result of the new English governess who had begun caring for the children: she was known to enjoy a drink, she argued with the nanny, and with Sergei, who sided with the latter whom he held in great esteem. This disruptive aspect of his personality lasted until he was around 8 years of age.

Freud was puzzled by this reported change and wanted to understand what was at stake for the child. He discovered that there were several irrational fears and rituals evident in childhood. Sergei developed a fear of wolves and was teased by his sister who would upset him with an illustration of the animal from a book. But this fear was not limited to wolves; beetles and caterpillars also became a source of anxiety for him. Freud recounted one occasion when the child was pursuing a butterfly and, while doing so, became afraid of butterflies, forcing him to stop the chase. This fear of animals, which had emerged as he approached the age of 4, also puzzled Freud who learned that the boy had simultaneously taunted caterpillars, cutting them into pieces, and was violent towards horses, without fearing them (Freud 1918b, 211–215).

Up until the age of about 10, Sergei also became unusually zealous in his religious worship and developed a nightly routine of praying and kissing any icons in the house (p. 260). Blasphemous thoughts entered his head, and a strange association occurred: the sight of horse manure in the road would result in the thought that *God is shit* (pp. 267, 281). He also experienced the fear of turning into the ageing men or beggars whom he passed in the street and created a ritual of breathing out in an exaggerated fashion as he passed them.

Freud wanted to understand what the impact of the child's relationship with his parents, sister and the governess had on these unusual behaviours. Relations between the governess and Sergei had initially been difficult. She insulted his nanny, and the child took the nanny's side. But had this been the cause of his anxieties?

Freud believed the child had developed castration anxiety, a fear of the violent loss of his penis in phantasy, as a result of numerous childhood events. Firstly, he had recalled the governess giving him chopped sugar sweet sticks, which she had described as resembling snakes that had been cut up (p. 240). Sergei had also been told the story of Reynard, a cunning mythical fox who lost his tail in the ice while using it as hunting bait. Freud also identified the importance of the boy witnessing his father chopping a snake into pieces when out walking as a possible source of this irrational castration anxiety (p. 240), which may have led to his fear of horses and caterpillars, owing to their phallic shape. But, above all, it was a dream that unravelled the mysteries of the child's obsessional behaviours.

The Dream of the Wolves

Here is the childhood dream, remembered in analysis, from the night before Sergei turned 4 years old:

> I dreamed that it is night and that I am lying in my bed (the foot of my bed was under the window, and outside the window there was a row of old walnut trees.

I know it was winter in my dream, and night-time). Suddenly the window opens of its own accord, and terrified, I see that there are a number of white wolves sitting in the big walnut tree outside the window. There were six or seven of them. The wolves were white all over and looked more like foxes or sheepdogs because they had big tails like foxes and their ears were pricked up like dogs watching something. Obviously fearful that the wolves were going to gobble me up I screamed and woke up. My nurse hurried to my bedside, to see what had happened. It was some time before I could be convinced that it had only been a dream, because the image of the window opening and the wolves sitting in the tree were so clear and lifelike. Eventually I calmed down, feeling as if I had been liberated from danger, and went back to sleep.

(Freud 1918b, 227)

The dream was described by "the Wolf Man" in slightly different ways on different occasions (Gardiner 1971). He also painted it. Freud argues that the dream – as a disguise – is full of reversals. First, the manifest dream reverses many of the latent dream-thoughts:

- It reverses the position of the wolves in relation to the tailor, a terrifying story told to Sergei by his grandfather – whereas in the latent content the tailor is in the tree and the wolves are below – a story young Pankejeff knew well.
- It gives the wolves big tails – whereas the latent content features tails falling off.
- It makes the child the object being looked at – whereas the latent content features themes of looking.

Freud asks if the dream-work is reversing so much of the latent content, could the stillness of the wolves in the manifest dream also be a reversal? Freud then constructs this reversal. He gathers together the elements of the dream along with other case material to make an extraordinary inference: the dream touched on an earlier memory of witnessing his parents having sex when he was 18 months old. Freud theorised this scene was the root of the obsessional neurosis (Freud 1918b, 234–241).

Let us take this seriously and consider Pankejeff first as a neurotic, as an obsessional. How was this invention derived, and what questions and contradictions arose in relation to this diagnosis given to him by Freud? Let us first begin with the diagnosis. *Obsessional* is one of two possibilities under the rubric structure of neurosis. Freud's original term, *the neuro-psychoses of defence* (Freud 1894), was shortened to *psychoneuroses*; it embraced not only hysteria but also defence psychosis, anxiety neurosis (phobias, traumas), states of paranoia, and obsessional thoughts and behaviours. Although Freud followed the psychiatry of his day and focused on symptom patterns, he quickly turned to explanations and to theorising the roots of neurosis and the mechanisms of his cures. His ideas about neuroses became intertwined with and inextricably linked to the development of psychoanalysis itself (Laplanche and Pontalis 1973, 226–227).

We find Freud far into this trajectory when he meets Pankejeff. Freud by then has created a treatment for neurosis and not for psychosis. Pankejeff does not present as psychotic. Freud relies not only on the initial symptoms to guide his diagnosis, but also on his own theory. In short, Pankejeff becomes a test case for Freud, a way to test his dream theory, the origin of neurosis in early childhood, and something new: the use of constructions by the analyst as a form of treatment. In this case study, Freud is also speaking back to Alfred Adler and Carl Jung, claiming the primacy of early sexual experience in the psychogenesis of neurosis. This case study is a layered argument.

Obsessional neurosis was identified by Freud in connection with the psychological mechanism of obsession (*Zwangsvorstellungen*), in connection with compulsive ideas and acts. Through the Rat Man (Freud 1909) and the Wolf Man (Freud 1918a, 1918b, 1918c) cases, obsessional neurosis became part and parcel of the theory of psychoanalysis. For Freud, obsessional neurosis involved a false connection between a repressed actual experience and an insignificant idea, which then becomes uncontrollably and inexplicably compulsive (Laplanche and Pontalis 1973, 282). In the process of living with this primary defence, its details are active and known to the subject, and in this sense conscious. But because the ideas and acts have been disconnected from their origin, which remains repressed and unconscious, an obsessional can become very seriously impaired in his relationships, ability to work, and of course, in his sexual relations (Freud 1918b, 269). There was a constellation of obsessional symptoms that Freud observed across cases: irrational compulsions, anal sexuality, holding in faeces, very high ideals, and a critical, cruel super-ego that presents the subject as worthless, as waste.[1]

Let us turn to Lacan now to consider in another way Pankejeff's original diagnosis of obsessional neurosis. In the final chapters of his seminar on Anxiety, Lacan turns our attention to obsessional structure and asks, "by what paths excrement comes to take on its subjectified importance at the level of the human being", adding that it is via the Other's demand there comes to be a "whole economy of the function of excrement" (Lacan [1962–1963] 2015, 300). The child is typically presented with a demand regarding his faeces *to hold it in!* In holding it too long, faecal matter becomes fixed as part of his body. Following that, there's the demand to *let it out!* But letting go entails a loss, an absence, as well as an acquiescence to the demand. The switching demand leads to a response, to the development of ambivalence. Then there's the problem of what happens when he lets it go. Lacan calls it "a fine poo" but the child should not get into it or smear it. Rather, the child should try to "find substitutes to smear" (p. 302). But the child doesn't want the substitutes, so we get to the symptom, what Lacan calls the "yea-and-nay" (p. 302). In short, this is why Lacan will say "the subject is divided and ambivalent with respect to the Other's demand" (p. 303).

Lacan speaks of the metaphor of the gift as emanating from the anal realm and adds that "so far nothing has explained the obsessional's very particular dealings with his desire" (p. 305). He makes some striking observations about the obsessional's desire: anyone who has treated an obsessional realises that his fantasies do not lead to acts; in fact, he conditions postponement as an enactment of his desire. Lacan locates this desire as a desire to create impossible desires. The result is that "whatever [the obsessional] may do to realise [desires], he doesn't get there" (p. 306).

In a chart presented in the first meeting of the year of the seminar, Lacan highlights the term "turmoil" (p. 13). Briefly turning to the Wolf Man's dream, he explains that turmoil is where anxiety arises in a traumatic confrontation. Stating that "the subject yields to the situation" (wolves in the tree, staring) (p. 312), he proposes "yieldable objects", an object or objects that can become "equivalents" to the original. This "is a piece that can be primordially separated off [which] conveys something of the body's identity" (p. 314). The anal object "comes into play in the function of desire with this function of the yieldable object" (p. 315). But in the obsessional, desire is located at the level of "inhibition", and Lacan asks, "what is inhibition if not the introduction into a function ... of *another desire* besides the one that the function satisfies naturally?" (p. 316). He is speaking of the obsessional's desire to hold back.

For the obsessional, desire is a defence "that defends against another desire" (p. 318). What characterises an obsessional's behaviour? Compulsions. On the one hand, he cannot hold himself back and, on the other, when confronted with a task or advancement, he wavers, not knowing how to respond. Lacan reminds us that on both sides it is "the signifier that posits and effaces by turns" (p. 319). This illustrates the obsessional's endless search for satisfaction, a search that turns around and around on doubt. He doubts *all* possible objects that might substitute for a fixed ideal. Desire works as an active defence that drives a deadline back, so that the due date never arrives. The object *a* is excrement: excrement functioning as *a* which, as Lacan puts it, is "*a* as a stopper" (p. 320).

Let's turn now to the unconscious fantasy at play here. The idea of faeces as a gift becomes part of a *fantasy of oblativity*, seeing the gift as an offering. This unconscious fantasy has two sides: the subject gives to the other and sees the gift as an altruistic gesture, but "he expects to be loved as an image" as a result. The image is an *ideal of himself* which he maintains at a remote distance from himself, in the hands of the other(s). But as soon as the other questions the fantasy of the ideal image, the obsessional identifies as waste, becoming an object of no worth, thus impossible to love.

What is the end to such an analysis, with an obsessional analysand who is a master of postponement? Lacan declares, "at the very least ... he must realise that his desire is never allowed to appear in an act" and "that he sustains his desire at the level of the impossibilities of desire" ([1962–1963] 2015, 323). Let us leave Lacan here and return to Freud who adds a *variant* note to his Wolf Man case in 1918.

Here I refer to a brilliant study by Ilse Grubrich-Simitis (1996) titled *Back to Freud's Texts: Making Silent Documents Speak*. Strachey's translated and edited version of Freud's works is not the only version, nor is it the most accurate version! Freud's fair copy, written in his own hand, and variants which show what he crossed out and re-wrote tell us what Freud wrote and elaborated, wrote again and doubted, wrote and crossed out, changed. I do not read German and do not have access to the documents themselves. Nonetheless, what might we learn about Freud's thinking through these fair copies and variants concerning the Wolf Man? If we turn to the original manuscripts associated with writing this case history and consider what Freud was writing in the time delay between the ending of the case and its publication in 1918, one year before the Wolf Man returned for a short treatment, what contradictions and questions emerge?

Grubrich-Simitis (1996, 164) points out that when Freud discusses his patient's response to the reactivation of the primal scene, at the time of the nightmare when his patient was 4 years old, Freud adds a footnote:

> I may disregard the fact that it was not possible to put this behaviour into words until twenty years afterwards; for all the effects that we have traced back to the scene had already been manifested in the form of symptoms, obsessions, etc., in the patient's childhood and long before analysis.
>
> (Freud 1918a, 120, fn.1)

Of course, the above remarks are valid only subject to the condition of the reality of this scene as opposed to the assumption of its fantasised nature. A final variant made its way into the printed case: "It is a matter of indifference in this connection whether we choose to regard it as a primal scene or as a primal fantasy (Grubrich-Simitis 1996, 164).

At first glance, these two variants point to a contradiction of ideas. Contradictions in Freud's work as he is inventing psychoanalysis are neither unusual nor cause for alarm, in my mind. But there is additional evidence that Freud questioned himself regarding the status of the analyst's construction of the primal scene or primal fantasy. The case was ready for publication, but Freud delayed. He wrote to Sandor Ferenczi on 9 November 1914, soon after completing the case that he felt "cast into serious doubts" concerning the reality of the traumatic childhood experiences (p. 163). He was wondering if they were a matter of memories, of fantasies, or displaced combinations of both. He referred to the Wolf Man case as "the most delicate question in the whole domain of psychoanalysis" (p. 163).

While finishing the first draft of the Wolf Man case, Freud was immersed in writing *Totem and Taboo* (1913) and constructing there the murder of the primal father as a primal fantasy. He further elaborated the contradiction at the heart of his doubts in the twenty-ninth of the *New Introductory Lectures on Psychoanalysis* (Freud [1933] 1932). Freud elaborates the psychoanalytic concept of fantasy and explains that the fantasy of the primal scene can have the same pathological consequences as the actual observation of the primal scene (Freud 1918c, 216–253). A further crucial addition to the tools of treatment is Freud's technical article, "Constructions in Analysis" (1937), composed in response to criticisms of interpretations offered by analysts to their patients. The article begins with the question of evaluating the "yes" and "no" of the patient in response to an interpretation, and it considers the defensive value of negation. The goal of analysis is to expose repressed elements and enable the patient to experience reactions that may restore a forgotten past. To achieve this, the analyst has recourse to various indicators such as fragmentary and distorted memories that arise in dreams and ideas alluding to particular elements in order to offer a construction. What is crucial is the patient's response to the construction proposed by the analyst, beyond a yes, or a no. If the patient produces further material or if there is a change in the symptom, then the analyst can deduce that the construction was accurate by its effect.

Given these further writings, one might say that Freud grappled with the status of the primal scene/primal fantasy in the Wolf Man case for much of the rest of his life. Evidence of the power of fantasy to shape memory, "reality", and symptoms is by now accepted widely in psychoanalytic theory and treatment. I too accept this idea. But the question of the effect on the patient is crucial. Without this consideration of constructions in analysis, it is possible the analytic community will repeatedly reinstate and elaborate interpretations of the unconscious that do little more than defend the working theory of each of its practitioners. This positions the analyst as knower, as a master who emerges without the ethical compass of lack, ignoring the voice of the analysand as both guide and author of the analysis undertaken. It is this question of authorship that I will turn to next.

A Second Invention: Where Is the Subject?

I ask us to consider the Wolf Man as not only a most plausibly psychotic subject, but to consider what *psychosis is*, where the subject can be glimpsed, and how the real of the body and the imaginary ego are implicated in this structure in ways that are both pervasive and not always obvious. With this focus, I will present some of Lacan's comments on the Wolf Man in 1952–1953 prior to his third seminar on the Psychoses (Lacan [1955–1956] 1993), and also turn to some of Lacan's later work in the 1970s.

The notes I draw from here come from four talks Lacan gave in 1952–1953, early oral presentations and conversations with his colleagues. Lacan remarks on the Wolf Man:

> The Wolf Man is a person whose problems stem in part from what could be called an "uninserted" insertion into society. He presents a particular neurotic disturbance which had been described, before Freud saw him, as a manic-depressive state. For Freud there is no question of such a nosographical classification; what the Wolf Man presents should be considered as a state following on from the spontaneous cure of an obsessional neurosis.
>
> (1952–1953, 7)

I want to highlight "an 'uninserted' insertion into society" here, which I will return to later. Lacan goes on:

> Freud then published the Wolf Man as the history of an infantile neurosis. This childhood neurosis had a variety of manifestations … If you examine it

carefully, you see that what Freud's observations concentrate on is a detailed and passionate research, going one might say against the facts, into the existence or nonexistence of traumatizing events in earliest childhood.

(pp. 7–8)

In this way, Lacan calls into question Freud's construction of the Wolf Man's earliest experience. Then Lacan goes one step further:

What is an analysis? It is something that should allow the subject to fully assume what has been his own history. In the analysis of the Wolf Man, Freud was never able to obtain, properly speaking, the recall of the reality in the past of the scene around which the whole of the analysis of the subject nevertheless turns.

(p. 7)

In short, Lacan is saying that the interpretations of Freud do not move towards a history assumed by the Wolf Man. Lacan goes on,

History is a truth which has the property that the subject who assumes it depends on it for his very constitution as subject and history also depends on the subject himself since he conceptualizes it and then reconceptualizes it in his own way.

(p. 10)

In the case of the Wolf Man, for months and years the sessions produce nothing – this man speaks without contributing a thing, he is admiring himself in the mirror; the mirror is the listener, namely Freud on this occasion. Lacan also asserts:

His ego is a strong ego ... Not only does the Wolfman not succeed in assuming his own life. His instinctual life is "enclosed", "encysted": everything of the instinctual order comes on like a flood if he encounters a woman using a cloth to wash the floor, or a brush, and showing her back and her bottom.

(p. 11)

I presume Lacan means the ego is strong in the imaginary. Here Lacan evokes an encounter with the real that affects the body of the Wolf Man like a flood. Something of the ego repeats as a mirror, according to Lacan, and the Wolf Man is beset with a flood of bodily responses through chance encounters, as outlined in the quote above. I want to mark this moment because it says something about structure as it involves the ego and the body, and it points towards psychosis.

Indeed, a few years after finishing psychoanalysis with Freud, the Wolf Man stood in a street staring at his reflection in a mirror, convinced that some sort of doctor had drilled a hole in his nose. He had entered a new analysis with Ruth Mack Brunswick, a Freudian, who explained the delusion as a displaced form of castration anxiety, maintaining Freud's diagnosis and interpretive rubric (Gardiner 1971). Lacan also centred on the father in his remarks but connected the delusion of this street scene to the Wolf Man's persistent passive stance. He writes, "In the last phase of the illness one can see different types of paternal relationships being incarnated. Dentists and dermatologists are two very different series of personages" (Lacan 1952–1953, 22). Dentists extract teeth and the more they extract, the more the Wolf Man, according to Lacan, distrusts them and entrusts himself to them (p. 23). Dermatologists represent:

> fathers who are death-bearing on the plane of the most primitive imaginary relationship, in face of whom the ego of the subject flees and hides itself in a sort of panic. This type is linked to the image of the primal scene: it identifies the subject with that passive attitude, which is the cause of his most extreme anxiety, because it is equivalent to primal fragmentation … For the Wolfman the nose is an imaginary symbol: the hole that everyone else can see.
>
> (Lacan 1952–1953, 23)

Lacan then builds a picture of a crisis that emerges in the Wolf Man's analysis with Ruth Mack Brunswick. She works to dismantle the Wolf Man's position as:

> Freud's favorite son … Ruth Mack Brunswick shows him that Freud is not interested in his case. The subject then behaves like a lunatic. Freud appears immediately afterwards in a spectacular dream. The dream of the sick father looking like a begging musician. It is a mirror dream. The father is himself and Freud against whom he is making his complaint … It is a reassessment of all the relationships he had with Freud, and these relationships are … essentially aggressive. The subject is now at the height of his disorder.
>
> (Lacan 1952–1953, 25)

According to Lacan, this crisis is a turning point towards "reality". Yet it hinges on the Wolf Man establishing his own meaning. Here is Lacan again:

> The core of the problem is "his own meaning", namely the wolves. In a dream the instinctual origin of his troubles is on the other side of a wall at the end of which is found Ruth Mack Brunswick. He is on one side, the wolves on the other: it is the symbolization of the role that his desire has in determining his psychosis, that his desires should be recognized by the other and therefore find a meaning.
>
> (Lacan 1952–1953, 25)

Let me take this idea of the meaning of the Wolf Man a bit further. Both Freud and Lacan understand a delusion as a work of repair on the part of the psychotic, a repair that is stabilising. But what is teetering, so to speak, before that point? What is it that is repaired? How well does the repair work? While Sergei Pankejeff may be said to be stabilised with respect to madness or bouts of paranoia, the question remains about what has been repaired through psychoanalysis, and what still teeters even at the end of his life. Exploring these questions involves again considering psychosis as a structure, what psychosis is at its heart. The terms I explicate and develop below pertain to psychosis as *a structure* – a structure that creates a new social link for humanity. I will also return to the Wolf Man in relation to the problematic of inventing him at the end of this chapter.

Working with Cormac Gallagher's translation of Lacan's twenty-third seminar, *Joyce and the Sinthome* (1975–1976), I want to highlight four points of orientation in psychotic structure:

1 The ego ruptures into an open form that divests itself of the body and its affects.
2 The ego has enigmatic functions; it *is* the unconscious, and the unconscious becomes accessible through "the error" of epiphany.
3 When *jouissance* invades the entire body, it disorganises the subject and brings him close to the object that was not extracted, and this problematic must be treated by the psychotic himself.
4 The *sinthome*, illustrated through the typology of a Borromean knot, becomes a know-how with one's symptom. The *sinthome* also creates a singular *jouissance* and forms a new social link.

First, I'll unravel these four points through Lacan's last lesson of Seminar 23, and then provide a very brief exegesis of how they work in various writings by James Joyce. In this 1975–1976 seminar, Lacan creates a new topology to describe psychotic structure, showing how a fourth term added to the Borromean knot of the orders of the real, symbolic, and imaginary allows the subject to cohere when any of three orders may become disconnected. I will not go any further into this as that is beyond the scope of what I want to say here. However, throughout this seminar and especially towards the end of it, Lacan describes characteristics of psychotic structure that are striking in their implication for how we think of psychosis and its possibilities.

Lacan speculates that in psychotic structure, the ego is not in the form of a circle but has opened itself to the real. The open form of the ego is far from a liability. It is a form that veers from the illusion of a bounded whole firmly connected to a body image which, for Lacan, is an illusion to which the neurotic succumbs. Lacan tells us that Joyce can detach from his body, his body is "to be shed like the skin of a fruit" (Lacan 1975–1976, Lesson XI, 10); he has a body "like a piece of furniture" (Lesson XI, 16). The self, body, and ego are not unified; in fact, the body slips from this purely imaginary unity and frees itself of the imaginary; the ego is open to the real and remains open. The open ego, with access to the real, has an enigmatic function. In this function, Lacan tells us, the ego *is* the unconscious. Lacan takes a step away from the unconscious as structured by signifiers (of the symbolic) and declares, "One thinks against a signifier … One leans against a signifier in order to think" (Lesson XI, 18).

How does Joyce think? He thinks through encounters with his errors. Lacan argues that for Joyce "epiphanies are all always characterized by the same thing

… an error" and "the unconscious is linked to the Real … thanks to the mistake" (Lesson XI, 17). The subject leans into this problem with language: he finds enigmas, and his unconscious produces epiphanies which, in turn, read as indecipherable. He also lives with the problematic that *jouissance* invades the entire body, disorganises him, and brings him close to the void, and this problematic must be treated by the psychotic himself.

These then are the coordinates of a life structured by psychosis from the last works of Lacan: psychosis may be lived outside madness through an open ego; the unconscious is a function of the ego and is lived through riddles as well as a curious detachment from the body; and the subject transforms an invasive disorganising *jouissance* into a new construction, the *sinthome*. The *sinthome* is a fourth ring, an invention by the subject. For Joyce, it was the invention of a new form of writing used to stabilise the three rings of the real, imaginary, and symbolic. In Seminar 23, Lacan does not follow his former logic of making neurosis the primary structure and psychosis as produced by the foreclosure of the Name-of-the-Father. The Name-of-the-Father is a metaphorising process whereby a signifier, the father's signifier, is substituted for another signifier, that of the Other's desire, causing the subject to become organised by and subject to the signifier. Neurosis is re-considered thus as a special case created by the introduction of a specific signifier. Psychosis is structured by the foreclosing of the Name-of-the-Father. The delusion of psychosis is *one* response to this foreclosure; the symptom-metaphor of neurosis is another. The Oedipus complex is now a symptom.

Lacan demonstrates that the symbolic, the imaginary, and the real are linked like the rings of a Borromean knot – in such a way that severing any one link will untie the other two. This explains the triggering of psychosis as madness. Joyce succeeded in avoiding the onset of psychosis through his writing, which thus plays the role for Joyce of a *sinthome*, a fourth ring. A *sinthome* in this respect is an identification with a symptom and is a solution similar to that offered by the paternal metaphor. It organises the real of *jouissance* but does not make use of interpretation as would a signifier.

Lacan locates the elementary phenomena for Joyce alongside the experience of enigma in Joyce's "epiphanies". fragments of actual conversations overheard, extracted from their context, and carefully recorded on separate sheets. All his life, Joyce wrote what he heard and saw, and many of the fragments were subsequently reinserted unannounced into later texts such as *Finnegans Wake* (Joyce 1939). Torn from their context, the epiphanies remain nonsensical or enigmatic fragments and are striking for their qualities of incongruity and insignificance. While Joyce never experienced psychosis as a form of madness leading to hospitalisation, and he avoided the onset of psychosis through his writing which functioned as a *sinthome*, Pankejeff's life follows a very different trajectory: he experienced madness as hallucination, as paranoia, and he remained in treatment for six decades.

Where is the speaking subject? Speaking to what desiring Other? We ought to know something of his experience, no? Writing his memoir near the end of his life, the Wolf Man produces a delayed contribution, his part concerning a book about him, which he holds back until a deadline for publication looms. He put off any written contribution to the book, *The Wolf-Man by the Wolf-Man* (Gardiner 1971), until just prior to its publication. By then, he's been undergoing analysis for six decades, despite Freud's pronouncement of his being "cured", making him one of the longest-running famous patients in the history of psychoanalysis. *The Wolf-Man by the Wolf-Man* presents Freud's case history, notes from Ruth Mack Brunswick, an introduction by Anna Freud, as well as the Wolf Man's contribution of his memoirs.

The curious thing is that the memoirs read for me as a social history – a dry, detached history, the bare facts – and the reader can scarcely credit that its author has undergone any form of psychoanalysis. He has little to say about his subjective life. He does not take a clear stance; rather he both upholds and contradicts some details of his analysis with Freud. But mostly he presents an idealised picture of Freud. Thus, he finds himself writing about himself by not saying where he stands, what he thinks, or what he experiences. He is, in short, an object of psychoanalysis, over-written by psychoanalysts. Is this a suppletion? A suppletion supplements the paternal function when it is lacking. A substitute for the Name-of-the-Father? In other words, is this a form of writing *without saying* – a way to find a name in a wider social link that will assure him a place in history? Does it function as a *sinthome*, beyond an extension of psychoanalysis as a patient of the Father of psychoanalysis: Freud? The *Wolf-Man by the Wolf-Man* allows Pankejeff to take his place in psychoanalytic history, formed by the theory that gives him a name and a place. Yet as a speaking subject, particularly a subject of his own meaning, the Wolf Man leaves us with very little.

There is, however, the famous wolf dream, which Lacan returns to in his eleventh seminar in "Tuche and Automaton". He claims that the Wolf Man's dream is not a repetition of a scene, which would be always veiled in analysis through transference. Rather, it is a traumatic encounter with the real which cannot be symbolised and it terrifies the child and wakens him (Lacan [1964] 1998, 54–55). If we consider how the Wolf Man lived with this real, we may come to see that at some moments, he invented a way, in speech and in painting, to tame the real, to some extent.

And what of our own inventions of him? We have no access to the subject himself and, lacking that, we create versions of him to answer the problems of our time, for our patients. This is how I hear and honour the inventions of Freud, Lacan, and my colleague, Rik Loose (see Chapter 10).

Note

1   I use the masculine pronoun here because there is a masculine tendency to obsessional neurosis although it can affect both sexes.

References

Freud, Sigmund. (1894). "The Neuro-Psychoses of Defence". In *The Standard Edition of the Complete Psychological Works of Sigmund Freud*, translated by James Strachey, vol. 3, pp. 45–68. London: Hogarth, 1955.

Freud, Sigmund. (1909). "Notes on a Case of Obsessional Neurosis". In *The Standard Edition of the Complete Psychological Works of Sigmund Freud*, translated by James Strachey, vol. 10, pp. 155–249. London: Hogarth, 1955.

Freud, Sigmund. (1913). *Totem and Taboo*. In *The Standard Edition of the Complete Psychological Works of Sigmund Freud*, translated by James Strachey, vol. 13, pp. 1–162. London: Hogarth, 1955.

Freud, Sigmund. (1918a). "From the History of an Infantile Neurosis". In *The Standard Edition of the Complete Psychological Works of Sigmund Freud*, translated by James Strachey, vol. 17, pp. 7–122. London: Hogarth, 1955.

Freud, Sigmund. (1918b). *Wolfman and Other Cases*, translated by Aday Huish. London: Penguin Books, 2002.

Freud, Sigmund. (1918c). "From the History of an Infantile Neurosis [The 'Wolfman']". In *The Penguin Freud Reader*, edited by Adam Phillips, pp. 196–309. London: Penguin Books. 2006.

Freud, Sigmund. (1933 [1932]). "Lecture XXIX: Revision of the Theory of Dreams". New Introductory Lectures on Psychoanalysis. In *The Standard Edition of the Complete Psychological Works of Sigmund Freud*, translated by James Strachey, vol. 22, pp. 7–30. London: Hogarth, 1955.

Freud, Sigmund. (1937). "Constructions in Analysis". In *The Standard Edition of the Complete Psychological Works of Sigmund Freud*, translated by James Strachey, vol. 23, pp. 257–269. London: Hogarth, 1955.

Gardiner, Muriel (ed.). (1971). *The Wolf-Man by the Wolf-Man*. New York: Basic Books.

Grubrich-Simitis, Ilse. (1996). *Back to Freud's Texts: Making Silent Documents Speak*, translated by Philip Slotkin. New Haven, CT: Yale University Press.

Joyce, James. (1939). *Finnegans Wake*. London: Penguin.

Lacan, Jacques. (1952–1953). *Notes on the Wolfman*. In *The Seminar of Jacques Lacan*. Unknown translation from unedited French manuscripts. Retrieved from https://lacanianworks.net.

Lacan, Jacques. (1955–1956). *The Psychoses*. In *The Seminar of Jacques Lacan, Book III*, translated by Russell Grigg, edited by Jacques-Alain Miller. London: W.W. Norton & Co. 1993.

Lacan, Jacques. (1962–1963). *Anxiety*. In *The Seminar of Jacques Lacan, Book X*, translated by Adrian Price, edited by Jacques-Alain Miller. Cambridge: Polity, 2015.

Lacan, Jacques. (1964). *The Four Fundamental Concepts of Psychoanalysis*. In *The Seminar of Jacques Lacan, Book XI*, translated by Alan Sheridan, edited by Jacques-Alain Miller. London: Penguin, 1998.

Lacan, Jacques. (1975–1976). *Joyce and the Sinthome*. In *The Seminar of Jacques Lacan, Book XXIII*, translated by Cormac Gallagher from unedited French manuscripts. Retrieved from http://www.lacaninireland.com.

Laplanche, Jean, and Pontalis, Jean-Bertrand. (1973). *The Language of Psychoanalysis*, translated by Donald Nicholson-Smith. New York: W. W. Norton.

Chapter 10

The Wolf Man and Psychosis in the Post-Oedipal Era

Rik Loose

Introduction

Freud's Wolf Man case study is complex and convoluted. Freud and indeed many others have over-interpreted and over-constructed the case. It does not reflect how we practise psychoanalysis today, at least not within the Lacanian orientation since Lacan, as psychoanalysis has undergone a big evolution, as "clarified recently by Jacques-Alain Miller" (Demuynck 2016, 134). Indeed, psychoanalysis today moves in a direction which runs counter to an over-abundance of meaningful inter-pretations and constructions. The case of the Wolf Man is the first time that Freud extensively refers to constructions in analysis (Freud 1918, 50–51) when, based on the dream that gave the Wolf Man his name – a point not without importance, as we will see – Freud constructed a *this-is-what-must-have-happened* of the *primal scene*, which Freud proposed on the basis of his patient's observation of the *coitus a tergo* of his parents when he was a year and a half. Reading the case, we get the impression that Freud is hunting something down or he is imposing himself on the case which surely was not without effect, like imposing the name of Wolf Man on his patient, Sergei Pankejeff. The latter may even have had a stabilising effect as the Name-of-the-Father was foreclosed, as we shall see. This does not mean that because of his involvement in a psychoanalysis he became a pacified and stable person, and it raises the question of whether this case was a failure. *An answer to this question is yes, but then*, as Freud tells us, successful cases do not teach us very much (Freud 1918, 10). Indeed, cases succeed, he says, at times quickly because everything that was needed was already known.

The case is difficult or frustrating to read because it is full of complexities, new questions, contradictions, speculations, and thus unfamiliar terrain. As Freud says, he wants "to bring forward some new facts for investigators who have already been convinced by their own clinical experiences" (Freud 1918, 13). This is important because in analysis it is not a good idea to *understand* the patient, but there is a tendency in most of us to do so when we are confronted with enigmas or aspects we don't understand. It is precisely at those moments that we should continue to listen and be taught by patients, rather than put all our effort into understanding. When we do that, we are not listening, and we hear nothing that can teach us

DOI: 10.4324/9781032663746-16

something. Understanding something implies that we are familiar with it and people tend to gravitate towards the familiar whereas what is not understood upsets the equilibrium that the familiar upholds. Hence, working as an analyst requires a certain amount of courage. To this point, Miller says: "[t]his reading [of the Wolf Man case] really is only of interest if we suspend our acquired knowledge" (Miller 2010b, 43). He continues by saying that we could read this case on the basis of "trying to learn what neurosis and psychosis are … taking as your starting point the principle that you don't know what they are" (Miller 2010b, 43). This concerns "approaching an analytic case by forgetting what is already known … learning what psychoses, neuroses and perversions are from the basis of what a subject says about it" (Miller 2010b, 43).

This is not easy when the articulations of the Wolf Man have been drowned in so many interpretations and constructions. Yet this is what we must do. In "Inhibitions, Symptoms and Anxiety", Freud writes: "[i]t is almost humiliating that after working so long, we should still be having difficulty in understanding the most fundamental facts" (1926, 124). Miller comments about this, saying:

> this affect of near shame brings together the dignity of the work that we carry out, which is to confront us with the most fundamental data of analytical experience and theory, and which at times makes us perceive that we don't manage to grasp them.
>
> (2010b, 74)

He continues by saying that this is particularly relevant as the concept of castration plays such a crucial role in this case. This is not clear in the case. Freud introduces here the term *rejection* (*Verwerfung*) of castration. Lacan uses this term and turns it into *foreclosure* as the fundamental mechanism for psychosis. Castration may well be a fundamental Freudian concept, but do we really know what it is? Did the Wolf Man accept castration?

Our approach will be to learn something from some of the questions, confusions, complexities, and paradoxes of this case to say something about psychosis today. A limited number of elements of the Wolf Man case will form a starting block in plotting a course that will also allow us to consider aspects of psychosis today. For a detailed analysis of the case, the reader is referred to Miller's articles, "The Wolf Man I" (Miller 2010a) and "The Wolf Man II" (Miller 2010b). These are exhaustive accounts of Lacan's thinking on psychosis. Many books and articles have been written on this subject such as Stijn Vanheule's (2011) *The Subject of Psychosis: A Lacanian Perspective*. In what follows, I will extract aspects of the Wolf Man case to illustrate how the ideas that have been developed in the Lacanian orientation on psychosis, including those that have been consequential about psychosis in Lacan's later work and especially in his twenty-third seminar on the *Sinthome* ([1975–1976] 2016), allow us to reread the case of the Wolf Man as a case of psychosis. Arguably, had these ideas been available at the time, it could have led to a better treatment. These considerations will also allow us to illustrate some clinical aspects of the experimental idea of ordinary psychosis developed by Miller towards the end of the 1990s which lifts our thinking and treatment of psychosis firmly into the twenty-first century.

Castration and Foreclosure

Freud interpreted the case of the Wolf Man thinking it was a case of obsessional neurosis (Freud 1918, 22). What distinguishes a neurotic structure from a psychotic one is the acceptance of castration, castration-anxiety being the motive force for repression.[1] However, despite castration being a quintessential Freudian notion, it is, according to Miller, "not too clear in Freud" and he argues that Lacan attempts to clear it up (2010a, 9). To illustrate Freud's confusion, let's consider a passage from the Wolf Man case:

> He [the Wolf Man] rejected castration and held to his theory of intercourse by the anus …, he would have nothing to do with it, in the sense of having repressed it … but it was the same as if it did not exist … We find good subsequent evidence of his having recognized castration as a fact. In this connection, once again, he behaved in the manner which was so characteristic of him, but which makes it so difficult to give a clear account of his mental processes or to feel one's way into them.
>
> (Freud 1918, 84–85)

The Wolf Man accepted castration but also rejected it and even in the sense that he recognised it, there was a resistance and a yielding to it (p. 85). That is confusing because there are, as Freud writes:

> two contrary currents that exist side by side, of which one abominated the idea of castration, while the other was prepared to accept it and console itself with femininity as a compensation. But beyond any doubt a third current, the oldest and deepest, which did not as yet even raise the question of the reality of castration, was still capable of coming into activity
>
> (1918, 85)

Freud resolves this contradiction by stating that this situation is characteristic of how things work in the unconscious (p. 79). Freud is not entirely committing himself to clarity here, however, and what has become clear is that Freud thinks that there is something that has not registered in the Wolf Man with regard to castration. He indicates in the enigmatic second sentence of this passage that there is behind the feminine attitude something that could become active. It is perhaps telling that Freud immediately follows this with the incident of the Wolf Man's hallucination of cutting through his little finger (p. 85). Freud tried to force this hallucination within a neurotic schema, which determined the direction of the treatment, by interpreting this event as an example of the acknowledgement by the Wolf Man of the reality of castration. However, it is also clear in the quote above, ("He [the Wolf Man] rejected castration …") that Freud believed in the Wolf Man's rejection of castration by referring to the anal theory of coitus. It is here that the Wolf Man's wolf dream can be introduced (p. 29). This famous anxiety dream is one in which the wolves who sit still in the tree in front of the window gaze at him. This gaze is crucial because he is seeing himself being seen and this is what causes his anxiety. It is an object, the object *a* of the *scopic* drive, and the Wolf Man is in the position of being the object of the gaze.[2] To be or to approach this object is a cause of anxiety. However, Freud analysed the dream on the basis that the Wolf Man must have seen something and constructed what he saw as a *coitus a tergo* by his parents; the famous primal scene that took place, or not. Freud also suggests that he may have opened his bowels at that moment, which may not be without importance, as we will see.

As suggested, for Freud, there was a connection between the rejection of castration and the anal theory of coition. Thus we could say that something was not symbolically registered with regard to sexual difference for the Wolf Man in so far as an element of reality was not acknowledged by him. How should we understand this? In his seminar on the Wolf Man, Lacan says: "He never had a father who either symbolized the father and incarnated the Father …" (Lacan 1952–1953, 28). A father who symbolises the father is a symbolic father; this is a father who symbolises the father of reality; the real and imaginary father of daily life. A few years later in his seminar on psychosis, Lacan ([1955–1956] 1993) introduces his concept of foreclosure, and this concerns the foreclosure of the symbolic father or the Name-of-the-Father which is installed in a metaphorical process. This is the paternal metaphor which allows the child to separate from the mother by being able to signify her desire (and *jouissance*) via the Name-of-the-Father, a signifier which metaphorises the mother's desire. This means that becoming a speaking-being entails a loss. In Freudian terms, the mother, as a love-object, must be given up and this opens up for the child a relationship to its own desire. This is what Freud referred to as the prohibition of incest and the threat of castration.

Lacan says that "the search for the symbolic father carries within it the fear of castration and that throws him back on the imaginary father of the primal scene" (Lacan 1952–1953, 28). Indeed, a primal scene may have happened in which the Wolf Man imagined all kinds of things about this man, his father, pumping away at the back of his mother. This scene, if it happened, could of course not be fully understood by an infant and could only have led to imagining things about it and its protagonists. In other words, the scene points to the Wolf Man as being not yet symbolically anchored or grounded in the symbolic, resulting in his propensity to being thrown back onto the imaginary plane. However, the question here is was he, or did he ever become, symbolically anchored? It is clear from Lacan's reading of the case that he was not symbolically anchored and the Name-of-the-Father (the symbolic father), as that agency that hooks the subject to the symbolic, was foreclosed.

What evidence do we have for this lack of a symbolic father who was not there for him? Freud writes that the Wolf Man's childhood was characterised by the absence of his parents. His mother was sickly and did not concern herself much with the children and his father was largely not present because of his depression (Freud 1918, 13). We must keep in mind though that most of what is articulated in this case is an imaginary reality. These may well form accurate descriptive indications, but the presence of a father-function cannot be observed, it can only be deduced from the articulations of the patient. In this regard, Miller says that the problem is not the presence of fathers as the Wolf Man had many father-figures. The problem is not that he did not have a relationship with his father but that he was so encumbered by it. Rather, the problem is that he suffered from fathers and father-substitutes all of his life; there is anxiety linked to the place of the father and thus the father-function had no pacifying effect on him. Indeed, anxiety was always there and he did not get appeasement from his castration anxiety (Miller 2010a, 52–53).

However, the Wolf Man did get appeasement from religion. Let's consider the following quote from the case:

> If he [the Wolf Man] was Christ, then his father was God. But the God which religion forced upon him was not a true substitute for the father whom he had loved and whom he did not want stolen from him.
>
> (Freud 1918, 66)

The Wolf Man always remained stuck in some way, he could not move on, especially in relation to his father with whom he had an imaginary relationship, and which included a sexual aspect, from what we can deduce from the case. For example, he envied his mother's position in the primal scene and had acquired "feminine impulses" (p. 78) and he "might obtain sexual satisfaction from him [his father]" (p. 101). Miller states "here the father continues to be a sexual object for the subject …" (2010a, 79). It is clear from the case that religion, which was introduced to him by his mother, was an attempt to appeal to symbolic pacification. The failure of this attempt resulted in his attachment to the previous problem, which is to say, the problem of anality (p. 79). To put this in Freudian terms, the sublimation of the drive via religion, which could have lifted the drive onto a symbolic plane, did not happen. Religion had no *symbolically* castrating effect on the Wolf Man and instead kept sending him back to anality and the imaginary plane. Freud made clear that this implied an imaginary identification as a woman with his mother (Freud 1918, 77–78).

A lot more could be said about this case in support of the Wolf Man's psychotic position and his subjective position being insufficient to respond to the real. Instead, I will refer to two elements suggested by Glenn Strubbe as prominent in the case and supportive of a hypothesis of psychosis, as well as being useful in identifying what the Wolf Man invented to prevent a triggering of psychosis, at least for long periods (Strubbe 2014, 311). These two elements are the anal object pertaining to money, and the gaze or scopic object pertaining to anxiety.

Solution via the Anal Object

Throughout the case, Freud emphasises the Wolf Man's anal-sadistic constitution and equates, here as well as elsewhere, faeces to money (Freud 1918, 72). Money was important for the Wolf Man in a peculiar way. He wanted to be known as rich (p. 73) and when his sister committed suicide, he experienced no mourning as an affect but was glad he would now inherit more money (p. 23). Lacan says in his seminar that what the Wolf Man got from his father was not symbolic but of the order of the *patrimoine*, this latter being that which is inheritable from the father's estate, as opposed to what is symbolically transmitted by the father-function (Lacan 1952–1953). Later, because of the war, he lost all his money, and this had an enormous effect on him (Strubbe 2014, 313). Freud began to collect money from the psychoanalytic community which was, according to Lacan, a major mistake and contributed to the triggering of his psychosis because it appealed to a narcissistic satisfaction (Strubbe 2014, 313). In other words, this gesture by Freud amplified the imaginary plane in the Wolf Man who was without recourse to any symbolic solution. Unlike Freud, there was for Lacan no doubt about the Wolf Man's diagnosis. In "The Function and Field of Speech and Language in Psychoanalysis", he writes the following:

> It is true that another factor comes in here, through which reality intervenes in the analysis—namely, the gift of money … In this case, the gift of money is reversed by an initiative of Freud's in which—as in the frequency with which he returns to the case—we can recognise his unresolved subjectivization of the problems this case left in abeyance. And no one doubts but that this was a *triggering* factor of the Wolf Man's psychosis …
>
> (Lacan [1953] 2006, 256; emphasis added)

Symbolically mediated solutions can only come about when the vehicle that allows the subject to step onto the symbolic plane is in place, namely the Name-of-the-Father, which is introduced as stated above via the installation of a paternal metaphor. Moreover, as explained earlier, for Lacan, the introduction of the subject into language causes the loss of a vitality or energy in the body that Freud related to the drive and Lacan to *jouissance*. The introduction of the signifier thus causes a mortification of the body, but this mortification is only partial because a certain amount of this lost vitality or *jouissance* can still be enjoyed, albeit in a limited way, via the object that is constituted as such by this loss. This object has a paradoxical status in Lacan's thinking in that it is at the same time related to a negative in the form of a loss, as well as to a positive in that it allows for the partial recuperation by the subject of some of this lost *jouissance*. As mentioned, Lacan called this object the object *a*, cause of desire. It is crucial that this object is lost or extracted, because if that extraction has not taken place, due to the foreclosure of the Name-of-the-Father, the subject is threatened by an overwhelming *jouissance* that is not limited. The subject will run the risk of being overwhelmed by an unlimited real *jouissance* against which they can defend themselves with delusions, hallucinations, or other inventions.

The Wolf Man had an odd relationship to money as an object. However, there are other odd or elementary phenomena – signs or symptoms that are indicative of a psychotic structure of the subject – discernible in this case. We can read that the world was hidden from the Wolf Man by a veil, but that when he passed a stool, for example, via an enema, he felt suddenly well and for a very short while saw the world clearly (Freud 1918, 75, 99). Defecation or the extraction of the object-faeces had become the condition for lifting the veil between him and the world. Then there were bodily phenomena such as intestinal problems, as in constipation, that Freud related to his mother when she exclaimed, when suffering from her own bowel problems when he was four and a half, "I can no longer live this way" (pp. 76–77). In this context, Freud is again referring to an (imaginary) identification with his mother and a problematic relationship with death. Moreover, there is the Wolf Man's sexual object-choice. This relates to the famous Grusha scene (pp. 91–94). Miller says that Freud leaves it till the end to mention it because it provides him with a solution to the case, namely, "there is in this subject a current of fundamental masculine identification which makes resolution possible" (2010b, 39) and whereas the primal scene places the Wolf Man in a feminine position, exacerbated by the seduction, the Grusha scene places him in a masculine position. Freud writes that the Grusha scene allowed him to win his way "to complete masculinity" (Freud 1918, 117–118) and from then on he was able to retain women as his sexual object, but this remained nevertheless problematic for the Wolf Man as illustrated by what Freud adds: "but he did not enjoy this possession …" and, as Freud writes on the previous page, the Wolf Man was in the grip off "a compulsively falling in love that came on and passed off by sudden fits" (p. 117). In the "Grusha scene", the Wolf Man saw a servant girl kneeling on the floor with a pail and a broom beside her. Grusha held the same posture as his mother in the primal scene, as he was seeing her from behind. From then on, a woman in this position will be destined to cause an infatuation in him that is overwhelming, invasive, and violent (pp. 91–94).

What is at stake here is an image of a behind in which the scopic and the anal are knotted but without any symbolic mediation (Strubbe 2014, 314). The symbolic element is missing, foreclosed. In an interview with the journalist Karin Obholzer (1981), Sergei Pankejeff became somewhat agitated after he had introduced his lover Louise into the conversation and said that women were only interested in money. He added that he kept giving her money without knowing why. He then indicated there were other women besides Louise and his wife Therese. He slept with them, gave them money when they didn't ask for it. Yet for him they were not prostitutes. He could have sex with them only when he gave them money. They seemed to be an enigma for him that he tried to resolve with money, and he had to be the one who gave it (Strubbe 2014, 316–317). For the Wolf Man, it was important that he gave away money. His symptom regarding money was not of an obsessional nature in the sense of wanting to hold on to money or retrieve it from the Other, nor indeed was it the compulsion to give it away as a reaction-formation against the former two. Rather, the Wolf Man had invented a symptom that functioned as a substitute for symbolic castration. This symptom allowed him to extract the object to create an artificial loss in what he experienced as too-much of *jouissance* in the real. As a result of the foreclosure of symbolic castration, at a fundamental level his object was not lost and so he was compelled to repeat his symptom of extraction. We can now understand why, according to Lacan, it was a mistake to give him money and why it may have destabilised him: the Wolf Man had no symbolic anchor and thus no experience of loss that made him desire.

Let's now turn our attention to the gaze in this case.

Solution via the Scopic Object: The Gaze

Miller begins the second part of his Lacanian analysis of the Wolf Man case by considering the gaze. In the primal scene, he is the one who gazes upon his parents. In the scene with Grusha, he gazes at her behind and he urinates. In this latter scene, the gaze triggered something that Freud thought to be erotic (Freud 1918, 93). However, there is the other perhaps more important aspect of the gaze; that is to be its object, to be seen. Miller says there is a drive in the Wolf Man to be seen and he is "stuck in the position of making oneself be seen" (2010b, 8). When he related his wolf dream to Freud, it became clear that there was something too much there for him, something that caused him anxiety and woke him up. The real was too much present and anxiety is a signal of the real. Freud suggested that a kind of reversal took place in the Wolf Man, going from the stillness or immobility of the wolves that looked at him to something he saw that was of the nature of a violent motion (Freud 1918, 35). According to Freud, what he saw was the primal scene. Then there is in the dream the sudden opening of the window which exposed the Wolf Man to the gaze of the wolves. In his seminar about the Wolf Man, Lacan says this window is a mirror in which the Wolf Man is seen to be seeing by the animals (Lacan 1952–1953, 17). In the moment the window opened, he became an object (of the gaze) and the window lost its protective function. From his analysis with Ruth Mack Brunswick, we know that he was very attached to images, especially those of himself and his mirror-image which pacified him. But when there was movement (for example, the sudden opening of the window) or a crack appeared in the image (such as the confrontation with Freud's face after his surgery for cancer), all hell broke loose (Strubbe 2014, 320–321).

There are more examples provided by Strubbe but what has been mentioned is sufficient to indicate that seeing and the drive to see protected him from the paranoia-inducing real invasion of the gaze; being seen, being the object of the gaze (Strubbe 2014, 320–321). A confrontation with this gaze caused a serious loss of his subjective consistency. Was the Wolf Man also here able to invent something to give himself some subjective consistency? From the interview with Obholzer, we know that Pankejeff was severely inhibited and everything he undertook came to very little. Strubbe indicates that the one exception to this was painting (2014, 323).

In Seminar 11, Lacan says that there is in painting a taming of the gaze (Lacan [1964] 1994, 109). In other words, painting can pacify the gaze as drive-object. Pankejeff became an avid and enthusiastic painter. This had become the solution he invented to counteract the paranoia emanating from an intrusive gaze from which he was not sufficiently protected. Psychotics often invent solutions as a response to a real that is too invasive.

Towards a Clinic of Psychosis Relevant for Modern Times

The Wolf Man case is endlessly fascinating. We keep coming back to it and opinions regarding diagnosis are divided. This case raises more questions than answers and this is a situation for psychoanalysis that is not without merit because it allows us to question established knowledge relative to some aspects of the Wolf Man's analyses with Freud and with others. Freud's treatment of the Wolf Man ended in 1914 and Freud regarded him as cured (Freud 1918, 121–122). In 1919, after the First World War, he went back to see Freud and later Ruth Mack Brunswick. He was a changed man, his obsessional symptoms had turned into somatic and paranoid complaints, and he experienced delusions of grandeur. Some analysts, including Freud himself, thought he was obsessional, others thought he was psychotic. Had the Wolf Man entered analysis with Mack Brunswick in the preliminary stages of psychosis? That may well have been the case, however, if he was psychotic, he did not suffer from a classic psychosis, such as was the case for Schreber (Freud 1911). There were no recurring visual or auditory hallucinations, no delusions on a grand scale, and no obvious language disturbances. If there were indications of psychosis, they were discreet (or subtle). A florid psychosis was not triggered and that sets us on the path towards a consideration of psychosis that is situated beyond the classic conception of it, one proposed by Miller as a hypothesis in 1998 and which he called ordinary psychosis. This conception has been further developed by analysts in the Lacanian orientation, taking as their point of departure Lacan's thinking on psychosis from the later period in his work. A seminal article on ordinary psychosis, its inception and how to diagnose it is Miller's (2009) "Ordinary Psychosis Revisited". A brief exploration of these ideas will allow us to say something about psychosis in modern times. This is a conception of psychosis that is situated otherwise than within the framework of the classic Oedipus complex.

For Freud, the Oedipal problematic turned around the function of the father. Lacan's initial innovation was to call this function the Name-of-the-Father and to emphasise that this function concerns a symbolic element. This element is something that must intervene between mother and child and if that does not happen, this Name-of-the-Father is foreclosed, and the paternal metaphor is not installed. The child remains caught in the enigmatic desire of the mother and is confronted without protection from the real of her *jouissance*. This classic Lacanian theory of psychosis is, as suggested earlier, generally well known in the psychoanalytic community. We assume that many readers are familiar with these ideas. Our wish is to give a glimpse of what it means to bring the clinic of psychosis into the twenty-first century. The idea that there is a Name-of-the-Father that supports, sustains, and creates order in the symbolic is no longer valid. Of course, there are some who, mostly for nostalgic reasons, want to hold on to this reassuring old order. However, clinical reality makes different demands, and we owe it to our patients to respond to these demands, not necessarily by giving in to them, but by being sufficiently informed about them and to be able to respond to them in a clinically relevant way.

We note that what dominates our culture, and thus our clinics, is not so much the dynamics of desire and lack but the dynamics of *jouissance* and the real. Towards the end of his work, Lacan had stumbled upon the concept of a real without law that could not be absorbed by the symbolic. In fact, absorbing the real was the great hope of the classic period of Lacan's return to Freud. Lacan began to accept the idea that all people, each in their own singular way, invent ways to respond to this real. People, including psychotics, invent things. The Wolf Man invented ways of extracting an object to cope with an overwhelming *jouissance* experienced by him as an imaginary veil between him and the world, with painting protecting him from an intrusive gaze.

People will always have to invent when language cannot do its work, and for the later Lacan, there is always a hole in language through which language is linked to the real. Consequently, language can never fully protect us against this real. People invent, and psychotics, like schizophrenics, must cope without having recourse to established discourse (Miller 2012, 254). They must invent something or some way of being able to use their bodies and organs. To a certain extent, that also applies to neurotics who respond to this real with their symptoms. If the symbolic contains a hole and thus the Name-of-the-Father is in deficit in relation to this hole (or real), then all kinds of things can be invented to make up for this deficit such as delusions, symptoms, activities, art, identifications, and so on. All these can function as substitute Names-of-the-Father. Put differently, the Name-of-the-Father is not the only way to provide some basis for the consistency of the subject by doing something with this hole in the symbolic. This clinic, based on the later Lacan, is quite pragmatic. Here, the treatment of *jouissance* – aiming at the singularity of each patient beyond the binary clinic of neurosis/psychosis – comes to the fore. The difference between the classic clinic of Lacan and the later clinic can be stated as follows:

The classic clinic is based on the idea that the Other (A) of language can absorb the real of *jouissance*. This represents Lacan's return to Freud which includes the idea that the function of the Name-of-the-Father can signify the desire and *jouissance* of the mother and provide the child with its own desire and subjective consistency. The later clinic is based on the idea that the Other contains a hole and thus everyone is confronted with a real without law (Laurent 2012, 246–247).

This made Lacan exclaim that "everyone is mad, that is, delusional" (Lacan [1978] 2013, 3). What Lacan meant by this comment is of course open to interpretation, but we can speculate that the clinic following Lacan's later work is a de-pathologising clinic and not a clinic of deficit, a clinic in which psychosis can be quite ordinary and creative. As already mentioned, the Wolf Man case is important because it raises many questions and challenges our established knowledge. Psychoanalysis as a theory and a practice should never be considered to have been fully finalised and must be considered to be in a continuous process of ongoing development. Indeed, there is little room for nostalgia in the Lacanian orientation, as a treatment can only properly take place when both analyst and analysand are open to surprise and to that which is new and not already established in advance. That is an absolute given in a field that orients itself around a central hole in knowledge, namely, that the question of what exactly a psychoanalyst is remains an open one, which implies taking up the position that an analysis must be invented in every case.

There Is No Guarantee and Some of Its Consequences

In his sixth seminar, Lacan announces the "big secret of psychoanalysis", namely, that there is "no Other of the Other" ([1958–1959] 2019, 298). The implication is that there is a lack in the Other because there is nothing that guarantees the symbolic order. In fact, logic does not permit that the truth of a system is demonstrated by an element – Name-of-the-Father – of the system. Where Freud shipwrecked himself on the "rock of castration", Lacan crashed into the real and the non-rapport of the sexual relation. These could not be absorbed or resolved by the symbolic as it contains a hole. This real kept on logically, clinically, and experientially raising its ugly head. For the real of the twenty-first century, Miller proposes that it is in great disorder because of the combined forces of science and capitalism (2013, 200). Times have changed as they always do and this has repercussions for people, how they suffer, experience madness, and how they respond to it. When language fails, the subject must invent something – irrespective of whether he or she is psychotic or not – to respond to this real and its disorder. What is crucial is that these inventions are not imposed on patients by the Other (the analyst). The Name-of-the-Father is one way of providing support for the subject to supplement the hole in language, but it is by no means the only way. Indeed, if the Name-of-the-Father is in operation, we can speak of neurosis. Increasingly, however, this Name-of-the-Father is not functioning. As a result, various things such as symptoms, inventions, or activities can function as substitutes for the Name-of-the-Father, or they operate as new Names-of-the-Father. Many of these can be discreet in the sense of being delicate or subtle (as opposed to discrete which emphasises that aspect which is distinct in an element), and if these "solutions" are new Names-of-the-Father, then in many cases we can speak of discreet signs of psychosis and neurosis as just one "solution" within a whole series of possible solutions. In the development of Lacan's thinking, the Name-of-the-Father loses some of its status. Does that imply that repression as the cause of neurosis has lost some of its power, bearing in mind that castration-anxiety is the cause of repression? It is not so difficult to observe this in our modern culture when we consider, for example, the constantly changing norms regarding *jouissance*, our increasing appeal to our rights to *jouissance* and consumption. In this sense, we are less inclined to hold back. The more traditional, symbolic ideals have lost some of their credibility and traction.

Therefore, it should not come as a surprise that the treatment of *jouissance* and the body – for *jouissance*, one needs a body – happens less via repression. The Freudian clinic and the classic clinic of Lacan were clinics of repression which implied that repression and its symptomatic return treated *jouissance*. The psychoanalytic acts were concerned with the productions of truth and meaning, and more or less left it at that. The modern clinic is more complex in that it concerns the treatment of *jouissance*, but only after having meandered through the layers of desire, truth, and meaning. In this modern clinic, the presence or absence of the Name-of-the-Father is less important than it once was. The question that guides the modern clinic is how, on a case-by-case basis, can *jouissance* be limited, localised, transformed, nominated, translated when it threatens to spread, become too much, or overwhelm the subject? What has come to the fore is a more continuous clinic in which it is recognised that the underlying discontinuity is formed by the radical singularity of the subject rather than by the discontinuity of the psychosis/neurosis binary. To use a cliché, the symbolic "is what it is" and if you believe in it, that may be helpful. However, if you are an unbeliever, your relationship to language and the Other is of an ironic nature. It means that you can see through language, see it for what it is, as nothing more than a semblant. This provides a different perspective, one that can be immensely creative. For example, James Joyce showed language for what it is, in essence, a material; the material that Lacan called *lalangue*. Let us now look at *lalangue* and language.

A Private Language

The existence and justification of language as a signifying system cannot, as we have seen, be supported by language itself. There is only one thing that can support it as a signifying system and that is, according to Lacan, that language is a material that has signifying qualities. However, that does not mean that this signifying quality is its first function. It only means that the material is there as a condition for it. For Lacan, this initial quality of language is that as a material, it is and causes *jouissance*; it consists of *jouissance* elements that are characteristic of the very beginning of language development in the child, which he called *lalangue*. We can observe it in very young children who enjoy words but, also, in those whose bodies can be traumatised by it. This *jouissance* has clearly little or nothing to do with meaning or communication. The first function and effect of language are to affect and traumatise a body. The babbling and speech-*jouissance* of children form a private language without communication and thus it does not create a social bond. This private language includes the rhythm of language, the rhythmic interactions that take place between child and Other. This rhythmic interaction is an absolute necessity – a necessary dance – that needs to take place such that the child can come to be in language. We should say that this concerns the rhythm of the signifier and is not something separate or prior to it. It is the drumbeat or percussion of language on the body.

Already in Seminar 3, Lacan proposes that prior to language proper there needs to be this kind of material that allows memory and historisation to come into being (Lacan [1955–1956] 1993, 156). Within and underneath this *jouissance*-causing material of language, we find the real. It is possible that, if operant, the Name-of-the-Father can regulate this real for the subject. The Name-of-the-Father, again, is that mechanism that both grounds language and transports the human subject into the symbolic order and it is through having access to this symbolic that the subject is able to limit, distribute, and regulate the real of *jouissance*. When not functioning or foreclosed, replacement Names-of-the-Father can fulfil the same role. Nevertheless, despite all these regulatory possibilities, the speaking-being is structurally not protected from this real. We are its dupe and foreclosed from it. This foreclosure is more radical, according to Lacan, than the one of the Name-of-the-Father and this foreclosure requires symptoms and *sinthomes*, psychotic or not (Lacan [1975–1976] 2006, 102). Here, Lacan indicates for the first time (as far as I know) that there are two forms of foreclosure, namely, the foreclosure of the real from the symbolic which applies to every human subject and the foreclosure of the Name-of-the-Father which pertains to those subjects who have a psychotic structure. The implication is that the psychotic subject is foreclosed from both the real as well as from language in its function of grounding human discourse.

The Changed Landscape of Madness: Ordinary Psychosis and Transference

Psychosis and neurosis today have been drowned in a series of symptomatic solutions that are all related to the real from which the subject is foreclosed. Indeed, psychosis is now more ordinary in that we are beginning to recognise its occurrence as being much more frequent (or normal) than we thought, but also in the sense that the description of its phenomenology approaches what comes across as ordinary signs and symptoms of pathology and neurosis. The changes in Lacan's thinking about language, *jouissance*, and psychosis are extremely important for the context of this changed landscape of madness but there are too many of them to explore here in detail. However, it may be helpful to mention a few of them. In Seminar 11, Lacan says that only in the absence of cause are effects successful ([1964] 1994, 128). It is not easy to get at what Lacan means here, but one way of reading it is that if the cause is gone, then the effects are on a merry dance which, as Lacan says, the cause would like to join (p. 128). This cause, here, is a reference to the object *a* that causes desire by virtue of being lost when we enter the domain of language or field of the Other. At that moment, something of *jouissance* is negativised. Lacan writes it as -φ. When the incorporation of language causes a lack of *jouissance*, it will cause a desire for more. When this object – as lack – does not function as cause, when there is no castration – as in the case of the Wolf Man – when it does not function as cause, *jouissance*-effects will be dancing in an unbridled way. As such, they can threaten the subject in subtle and not so subtle ways. These effects can show up via the body as was the case with the Wolf Man, but they can also show up in language, which, in Lacan's later work, is posited by him as containing *jouissance* and thus possibly *jouissance*-effects. These effects can be discreet or not so discreet. For example, language can run away with the subject as exemplified by a manic episode in which there are often no quilting-points in the speech of the subject. Or more discreetly, a signifier can contain an enigmatic *jouissance*. It is important to be sensitive to these discreet signs. A clinical example of such a discreet sign is articulated by an (ordinary) psychotic patient who said: "my ears clog up every time I have to be in a social situation precisely like what happens to your ears when a plane descends quickly in order to land." It became clear through the analysis that what was at stake in this discreet symptom was an opaque *jouissance* over which she had no control rather than being a physiological response that applies to all of us in certain circumstances.

In this regard, the object *a* does not function when it is not extracted. On various occasions, Lacan refers to this as the subject carrying the object in their pocket, and the implication of this is the subject does not suppose this object to be located in the Other. On this basis, it is understandable that the transference to the Other is problematic in psychosis. In transference-love, the supposition is that knowledge is in the Other, but also that the object *a* is located there. For the psychotic subject, this Other, for example, an analyst, does not possess this knowledge or object, and as a result, from the subject's point of view, the transference goes in the opposite direction – and thus we can speak of a *reversed* transference. This can lead to para-noia. Or the analyst, again, from the subject's point of view, wants something from the subject, such as love or hate, and that has implications for treatment. It requires a manoeuvre from the analyst that avoids the will of the Other. For example, in erotomania, the sexual will of the Other threatens the subject. The psychotic patient is the object of the transference of the Other and that means that the analyst must be present in a different way than in neurosis. They must avoid becoming a threat-ening Other and, for example, the analyst must avoid being too interested in the patient/analysand or in possessing knowledge and occupying the place where truth is located. Zenoni (2013) provides an excellent overview in respect of the analyst's orientation to the psychotic subject. It also means that the sessions, to avoid being an *agalmatic* and enigmatic object of transference, are conducted on a more con-versational basis. Indeed, sometimes the analyst supports moving from theme to theme to avoid potentially triggering moments in the conversation (Vander Vennet 2008, 193–194).

Private Language and Further Aspects of Treatment in Ordinary Psychosis

If the first encounter with language is not with language as meaning or communi-cation, it is also not initially an encounter with a system or a structure that trans-ports the subject into the social bond or discourse. Rather, it is an encounter with bits and pieces of language the child enjoys but which are also traumatising. As Lacan outlines in his later work, language is not just a signifying structure but is first a substance that is also real and contains *jouissance* which affects the child. This aspect of language (*lalangue*) originates from the linguistic dance that takes place between the first Other/caretaker and the child. This dance is not unrelated to interactions like feeding, toilet-training, holding, etc. It is a private and singular language permeated by the drive and libidinal investments that leave traces behind, all of which takes place outside the influence of social normalisation (Vander Vennet 2008, 195). What normalises is the social bond, carried by language with its laws, codes, and grammar which process this private language by lifting it into the social order and allowing the subject to function there (p. 195). This private language is part of every speaking-being and it provides everyone with something that singularly *ex-sists* in him or her. What happens in psychosis is that the mastery of normalisation did not sufficiently take place. A psychotic patient is often very attached to his or her private language. The question then becomes: how to conceive of the relationship between analyst and psychotic patient based on this private language? (p. 196). What follows are some of the ideas proposed by Eric Laurent (2012) and others:

1 It is important that a conversation about the problematic *jouissance* (located in the patient's body in the case of schizophrenia) or located in the Other (in the case of paranoia) takes place and this private language is conversed between analyst and patient. Indeed, analysts must inform themselves, for example, about where this *jouissance* is located, and in doing so, they are not unlike the student of the psychotic.

2 This private language is also a way or mode of *jouissance* and that means that where it becomes problematic or excessive, the analyst must displace, lessen, or name it.

3 Sometimes it is appropriate to translate this private language and *jouissance* such that it can function within the social domain. This can happen by naming it, but also, via punctuating speech and creating moments of meaning and/or coherence in the discourse of the patient.

4 It may be helpful to look for something that can allow for the knotting together of *jouissance*, signifiers, and imaginary identifications in such a way that *jouissance* can be stabilised. Creativity, art, and writing may find their place here for certain patients. James Joyce was able to stabilise the *jouissance* of his body by creating his own language with his singular style of writing. This is what Lacan called Joyce's *sinthome*.

5 It may also be the case that isolating certain signifiers in the discourse of the patient may help to organise problematic, overwhelming, and enigmatic anxiety-provoking elementary phenomena experienced by the patient.

It is crucial that all of this takes place on a case-by-case basis. The treatment of psychosis within the Lacanian orientation is not occupational therapy. Clinical decisions must be made on a continual basis and there is no protocol or handbook that can serve as a guide here. The overall idea regarding treatment is that one starts from the singular *jouissance* of the private language of the patient. Then the analyst allows the patient to take steps towards the social bond in such a way that the patient, who has remained too attached and invaded by his private language, can come to function in the social field of the Other. The post-Oedipal clinic of psychosis is a discreet clinic and perhaps a more difficult one because what often stabilises psychotic subjects are traits, habits, symptoms, identifications, and behaviours that come across as neurotic, but after careful clinical judgement may turn out to be discreet signs of psychosis. Coming to such a conclusion may be beneficial for the direction of the treatment. That is why it is an ethical imperative to inform oneself as a clinician about psychosis in modern times. As Miller (2009) explains, this discreet clinic requires a reading of subtle signs in terms of intensity, colour, and tone, which may represent disturbances at the level of the social, the body, subjectivity, disturbances of the most intimate sentiment of life in the subject. He says that at the level of the social, there may be disconnection from others; at the level of the body, there may be phenomena that are not a translation of what is repressed; and at the level of subjective disturbance, there may be an *undialectisable* emptiness (Miller 2009, 108). It may also take a more melancholic form in which subjects identify themselves as rejected objects, as waste of the Other. It may even be a vagueness that the psychotic experiences, a veil between the subject and the world – as we saw in the case of the Wolf Man.

Notes

1 For Freud, castration occurs during the Oedipal phase when the child experiences a threat that castration may result from loving the mother. This threat is the motive force for resolving the Oedipus Complex. For Lacan, castration has nothing to do with the fear of losing – or having lost – one's penis. Rather, for him castration concerns the subject's entry into language, transported there by the function of the Name-of-the-Father. This causes a symbolic separation of the child from the mother which entails a loss of (incestuous) *jouissance*, a loss that causes the child to desire and moves the child from the position of *being* the mother's imaginary phallus to *having* the symbolic phallus (that is, one's own desire).

2 The object *a* is a crucial Lacanian concept and its meaning goes through different stages in the development of Lacan's work. However, its meaning essentially comes down to the following: it is that which is lost qua *jouissance* when the subject undergoes symbolic castration by entering the field of language (see note 1). The moment of this entry is when the subject becomes a barred subject with an unconscious and with having his or her own desire that cannot be satisfied. The object *a* is thus not the object that the subject necessarily desires, but rather is the object (or loss) that *causes* that desire. This object correlates with Freud's objects such as breasts and faeces and to which Lacan adds the object gaze and object voice as causes of desire.

References

Demuynck, Joost. (2016). *Inleidingen in de lacaniaanse psychoanalyse*. Leuven: Acco.
Freud, Sigmund. (1911). "Psychoanalytic Notes on an Autobiographical Account of a Case of Paranoia (Dementia Paranoides)". In *The Standard Edition of the Complete Psychological Works of Sigmund Freud*, translated by James Strachey, vol. 12, pp. 1–84. London: Hogarth, 1955.

Freud, Sigmund. (1918). "From the History of an Infantile Neurosis" In *The Standard Edition of the Complete Psychological Works of Sigmund Freud*, translated by James Strachey, vol. 17, pp. 7–122. London: Hogarth, 1955.

Freud, Sigmund. (1926). "Inhibitions, Symptoms and Anxiety". In *The Standard Edition of the Complete Psychological Works of Sigmund Freud*, translated by James Strachey, vol. 20, pp. 87–174. London: Hogarth, 1955.

Lacan, Jacques. (1952–1953). "Notes on the Wolf Man". In *The Seminar of Jacques Lacan*. Unpublished English translation draft.

Lacan, Jacques. (1953). "The Function and Field of Speech and Language in Psychoanalysis". In *Écrits: The First Complete Edition in English*, translated by Bruce Fink, pp. 237–268. London: W.W. Norton & Co., 2006.

Lacan, Jacques. (1955–1956). *The Psychoses*. In *The Seminar of Jacques Lacan, Book III*, translated by Russell Grigg, edited by Jacques-Alain Miller. London: W.W. Norton & Co., 1993.

Lacan, Jacques. (1958–1959). *Desire and Its Interpretation*. In *The Seminar of Jacques Lacan, Book IV*, translated by Bruce Fink, edited by Jacques-Alain Miller. Cambridge: Polity, 2019.

Lacan, Jacques. (1964). *The Four Fundamental Concepts of Psychoanalysis*. In *The Seminar of Jacques Lacan, Book XI*, translated by Alan Sheridan, edited by Jacques-Alain Miller. London: Penguin, 1994.

Lacan, Jacques. (1975–1976). *The Sinthome*. In *The Seminar of Jacques Lacan, Book XXIII*, translated by Adrian Price, edited by Jacques-Alain Miller. Cambridge: Polity, 2016.

Lacan, Jacques. (1978). "There Are Four Discourses". *Culture/Clinic* 1 (2013), 3–4. https://doi.org/10.5749/cultclin.1.2013.0003.

Laurent, Éric. (2012). "Psychosis, or Radical Belief in the Symptom". *Hurly-Burly: The International Journal of Lacanian Psychoanalysis* 8, 243–251.

Miller, Jacques-Alain. (2009). "Ordinary Psychosis Revisited". *Psychoanalytical Notebooks: Ordinary Psychosis* 19, 90–115.

Miller, Jacques-Alain. (2010a). "The Wolf Man I". *Lacanian Ink* 35, 7–83.

Miller, Jacques-Alain. (2010b). "The Wolf Man II". *Lacanian Ink* 36, 6–85.

Miller, Jacques-Alain. (2012). "Psychotic Invention". *Hurly-Burly: The International Journal of Lacanian Psychoanalysis* 8, 253–268.

Miller, Jacques-Alain. (2013). "The Real in the 21st Century". *Hurly-Burly: The International Journal of Lacanian Psychoanalysis* 9, 199–206.

Obholzer, Karin. (1981). *Entretiens avec l'Homme aux Loups*. Paris: Gallimard.

Strubbe, Glenn. (2014). "De Wolvenman Vandaag". *iNWIT* 11, 309–325.

Vander Vennet, Luc. (2008). "Overdracht en Psychose: Een Conversatie als Smeedwerk". *iNWIT* 4, 186–208.

Vanheule, Stijn. (2011). *The Subject of Psychosis: A Lacanian Perspective*. London: Palgrave Macmillan.

Zenoni, Alfredo. (2013). "Orienting Oneself in Transference". *Psychoanalytical Notebooks: Psychosis Today* 26, 111–129.

JUDGE SCHREBER

Psychoanalytic Notes on an
Autobiographical Account
of a Case of Paranoia

DANIEL PAUL SCHREBER

Born 1842, Leipzig
Died 1911, Leipzig, Leipzig-Dösen psychiatric asylum

*Sculpting language into
his own image...*

Freud, Sigmund. (1911). "Psychoanalytic Notes on an
Autobiographical Account of a Case of Paranoia
(Dementia Paranoides)". In *The Standard Edition of
the Complete Psychological Works of Sigmund
Freud*, translated by James Strachey, vol. 12,
pp. 1–84. London: Hogarth, 1955.

DOI: 10.4324/9781032663746-17

The Form and Matter of Hallucinations in Schreber's Message Phenomena

Leon S. Brenner

Aristotle (1999) famously posits in his *Physics* that all physical entities are a composite of both *matter* and *form*, an idea commonly known as *hylomorphism*. Extending his hylomorphic perspective to the domain of artistic creation, in his *Poetics* (Aristotle 2017), Aristotle contends that beauty in art is the outcome of form superimposed on matter, specifically in achieving a harmonious equilibrium and symmetry between the two, thus resulting in an aesthetically pleasing and emotionally engaging artwork. Hence, in this paradigm, a poet imbues language, the chosen material, with form, while a sculptor shapes stone or wood, their selected material, in accordance with a desired form.

Along a similar vein, I will examine the manner in which psychotic subjects deploy their hallucinations in a manifestation of form imposed on matter. Leveraging their creative abilities and improvisational talents, many psychotic subjects discover the means to stabilise the psychotic process based on their *know-how-to-do* (*savoir-faire*) with language. Drawing on Lacan's interpretation of hallucinations, with special emphasis on the pivotal role they assume within the psychotic process, my focus will centre on Lacan's development of hallucinatory message phenomena as delineated in his paper, "On a Question Prior to Any Possible Treatment of Psychosis" (Lacan [1958] 2006), and chronicled by Daniel Paul Schreber in his memoirs ([1903] 2003).

Lacan's Theory of Hallucinations

Hallucinations are commonly identified with psychosis and most notably with schizophrenia. Indeed, they are among the decisive factors in the diagnosis of these psychiatric categories in the *International Classification of Diseases* (ICD) and in the *Diagnostic and Statistical Manual of Mental Disorders* (DSM). In these diagnostic manuals, hallucinations are characterised as perceptual experiences of objects or events devoid of any external source, such as hearing one's name being called by a voice that is apparently unheard by others (World Health Organization 2022). Defined thus, hallucinations are reduced to a disruption in the correlational relationship between a perceptual experience and the order of "objective" reality.

DOI: 10.4324/9781032663746-18

Consequently, when mainstream media, notably films, portray hallucinations, they place significant emphasis on disruptions which manifest in the perception of people, animals, objects, or patterns that are actually not there. An exemplary film portraying hallucinations associated with schizophrenia is *A Beautiful Mind* (2001). directed by Ron Howard. This film is a biographical drama chronicling the life of the mathematician, John Nash, who suffered from schizophrenia and experienced auditory and visual hallucinations throughout his life. The film's representation of these hallucinations is both realistic and chilling, illustrating their profound influence on Nash's personal and professional trajectory.

In his 1958 paper, "On a Question Prior to Any Possible Treatment of Psychosis", Lacan, paying particular attention to hallucinations, develops an alternative view of them. This framework diverts from traditional phenomenological and perception-based definitions of hallucinations and instead emphasises their linguistic structure (Lacan [1958] 2006, 445). Essentially, Lacan characterises hallucinations as extending beyond mere pathology to being meaningful subjective experiences. As will be explored, these experiences are facilitated by certain existential predicaments at the level of the signification of one's position in the world and vis-à-vis others.

Lacan's argument is with the traditional definition of hallucinations which he believes to be inadequate for several reasons. Primarily, this conventional definition fails to encompass the multifaceted and complex nature of hallucinatory experiences. Hallucinations manifest in various forms and can sometimes play a critical role in the life of the subject, often possessing significant meaning and even facilitating the subject's stabilisation. Accordingly, Lacan argues that hallucinatory experiences should not be dismissed as mere pathologies, but instead should be recognised for their potential value. He encourages psychoanalysts to closely scrutinise their analysands' hallucinations, examining the potential ways these phenomena can be harnessed within the analytical process.

Lacan's critique finds resonance with Maurice Merleau-Ponty's commentary on hallucinations in his book, *Phenomenology of Perception* ([1945] 1996). Merleau-Ponty, an influential French phenomenologist philosopher of the twentieth century, established that perception isn't a passive process, but an active, embodied one intricately entwined with our physical and cultural environment. Building up his thesis on perception, Merleau-Ponty deconstructs multiple contemporary theories of hallucination in his book, *The Visible and the Invisible* (1968, 389–402).

Echoing Merleau-Ponty's critique, Lacan argues that human perception cannot be simplified to issues pertaining to external objects stimulating the senses, thereby producing in the perceiver mental perceptions. This argument gains clarity when we consider hallucinations that yield perceptual experiences devoid of any external, measurable object (Lacan [1958] 2006, 446). If there isn't an external source, how does this perception come into being?

Merleau-Ponty provides an answer: the perceived and the perceiver are intimately intertwined. He insists that perception isn't grounded in measurable facts of the objective world, as the perceiver is inherently a part of what is perceived. In other words, his phenomenology of perception posits that the human body plays a pivotal role in shaping our perception, as opposed to being a mere passive receiver of sensory data. Merleau-Ponty's concept of *flesh* encapsulates this idea: it represents the indistinct and pre-reflective aspect of human embodied existence deeply connected with the world's materiality. In *The Visible and the Invisible* (Merleau-Ponty 1968), he suggests that the lived body and the material world exist in a dynamic and mutually constitutive relationship that cannot be simplified or separated, giving the world an internal logic beyond its "objective" composition.

Lacan concurs with Merleau-Ponty's assertion that the experience of hallucinations follows an internal logic. However, Lacan differs in his understanding of the source of this logic. Instead of Merleau-Ponty's concept of the *flesh* or a corporeal mode of being-in-the-world, Lacan maintains that this logic arises from a signifying structure ([1958] 2006, 450–451). In doing so, Lacan diverges from Merleau-Ponty's corporeal vitalism, suggesting that the experience of hallucinations should be understood not in terms of their sensory qualities but in relation to their role within a process of signification.

As a result, Lacan's approach goes beyond addressing hallucinations as a disorder of perception. He focuses on the ways in which hallucinations impact the subject, how they participate in the creation and interpretation of meaning (p. 447). Therefore, Lacan discusses hallucinations as unique perceptions that profoundly reflect the altered process of signification. As Vanheule highlights, for Lacan, the key aspect is not the object of hallucination but the effect it has on the subject's process of meaning-making (Vanheule 2011, 85).

In Lacan's understanding, hallucinations are primarily an expression of a signifying structure presented through various sensory modalities. This is why Lacan predominantly pays attention to the linguistic elements of auditory hallucinations: the words that the psychotic subject verbally hallucinates ([1958] 2006, 446). Thus, visual hallucinations, in Lacan's framework, are considered to comprise signifying units linked to images while tactile hallucinations are viewed as signifying units connected to sensations of touch. Lacan, however, argues that hallucinations, regardless of their sensory type, serve as carriers of meaning or signification in the psychotic's experience.

Daniel Paul Schreber's autobiography, *Memoirs of My Nervous Illness* (Schreber 1903), offers a profound testament to the range and intensity of psychotic experiences, making it a vital source for Freud's and Lacan's investigations into psychosis. A German judge in the late nineteenth century, Schreber underwent several psychotic episodes during which he experienced an array of vivid and deeply impactful hallucinations.

Schreber's auditory hallucinations involved hearing voices that interacted directly with him, sometimes commenting on his thoughts and actions. These voices seemed to emanate from diverse entities trying to inflict spiritual death upon him or convey divine revelations. His visual hallucinations included seeing images of God and angels, and he also spoke of a kind of divine or supernatural illumination. Additionally, Schreber reported somatic experiences which made him feel as though his body was undergoing transformation or being manipulated by super-natural forces. He grappled with a range of bodily sensations and emotional states that were challenging to articulate.

Taken as a whole, Schreber's rich and complex accounts of his hallucinations demonstrate the profound ways in which the psychotic process can shape one's subjective reality. These experiences are not isolated or meaningless, but rather deeply intertwined with his sense of self, world, and others.

Message Phenomena

In "On a Question", Lacan delves into Schreber's account of his hallucinations to extract a unique form of hallucination that he terms "message phenomena". These hallucinations are distinguished by their incompleteness – they are fragmented sentences and partial thoughts that seem to intrude on the subject from outside.

Schreber's memoirs provide numerous instances of these phenomena, which he describes as emanating from "divine rays" (1903, 28, 55). These "divine rays" assail him with unfinished phrases such as "Now I shall...", which he feels com-pelled to complete with a response like "...resign myself to being stupid" (p. 198). Schreber presents many other examples of this type of hallucination, such as:

> "You were to be...", "...represented as denying God, as given to voluptuous excesses".
> "I shall...", "...have to think about that first".
> "It will be...", "...done now, the joint of pork".
> "This of course was...", "...too much from the soul's point of view".
> "Lacking now is...", "...only the leading idea, that is – we, the rays, have no thoughts".
>
> (pp. 198–199)

In each of these cases, the hallucinations seem to prompt Schreber into a sort of dialogue or interaction, involving him in a strained effort to make sense or com-plete these fragments of language and thought.

Message phenomena, as characterised by Lacan, are hallucinated words or sen-tences that burgeon in moments of interruptions in the flow of speech and leave the subject in a state of anticipation for meaning. They occur at a crucial juncture, when the subject is implicitly introduced in the sentence in a grammatical sense (Vanheule 2011, 92). The anticipation lingers until the completion of the sentence, which typically attributes some quality or condition to the subject. This anticipa-tion of meaning, according to Lacan, imbues the final message with a heightened sense of enigma and significance. The longer meaning is suspended, the more pow-erful the final perceived message is for the subject (Lacan [1958] 2006, 447).

Important to note is that this process works in two directions. Schreber's hal-lucinations often took the form of sentences that were perceived as coming from an external source, which he then internally completed. Conversely, the process can also involve external voices providing the completion to one's own internal monologues. In both cases, the process of signification – the meaning-making process – is interrupted. This disruption sets into motion an intense quest for meaning, driving the pursuit of signification into high gear. The completion of the sentence, whether internally or externally generated, offers a form of resolution to this process, grounding the subject with a particular signification or meaning. The signification may be unique to the individual and their subjective experience, however, indicating the intensely personal nature of these phenomena.

In "On a Question", Lacan furnishes an instructive case study drawn from his own clinical practice within a psychiatric hospital setting and already briefly explored by him in his seminar on psychosis ([1955–1956] 1993). The case features a psychotic patient, whose experiences offer crucial insight into the signifying structure of message phenomena. This patient, a woman, was admitted to the hospital alongside her mother in 1955. The patient and her mother conveyed a pervasive sense of torment and threat, purportedly originating from their neighbours – a couple composed of a woman and her lover. At the outset, the neighbour had been friendly, visiting their home with a frequency that was initially welcomed but which subsequently came to be viewed as excessive. This overbearing presence eventually led to the patient and her mother becoming totally estranged from the neighbouring woman (p. 50). As a consequence, the neighbour's behaviour underwent a radical shift, morphing into hostility and menace. The patient detailed an illustrative instance of this threatening behaviour to Lacan, involving an unpleasant encounter with the neighbour's lover in their apartment building's hallway. During this incident, she alleges to have heard the man verbally abuse her by referring to her as a "sow" (Lacan [1958] 2006, 448).

Lacan observed that the woman had great difficulty voicing this term. It appeared that her utterance of the word "sow" introduced a level of confusion. The meaning of the term and the motivation behind the man's choice to deploy it were unclear to her. Despite further questioning, she remained unable to identify any basis for this insult. The derogatory comment was perceived as an inscrutable and odd intrusion, forcibly imposed upon her from an external source. Lacan therefore hypothesised that this was an example of a hallucination (p. 449).

In this instance, what is hallucinated is the man's utterance of the word "sow". This word constitutes a series of unchained signifiers that have become dislodged from their original signifying chain – whether preconscious or unconscious – and that reappear from without as a strange element, imposing themselves upon the subject. Due to the absence of contextualisation provided by the original signifying chain, these detached signifiers appear enigmatic and unsettling, as though they are coming out of nowhere.

An unchained signifier can sometimes be traced back to its original context. In doing so, its enigmatic nature can be mitigated, relieving its potentially distressing impact. Following this line of reasoning, Lacan employs this approach in the aforementioned case. He inquires what the woman had said to her neighbour in the hallway prior to the offending remark. She remembers she uttered the words, "I've just been to the pork butcher's..." (p. 448). This is a seemingly ordinary sentence that, nonetheless, remains incomplete. This utterance merely introduces the woman as the subject of the sentence but fails to expound upon its intersubjective function: specifically, the reason the woman would utter such a phrase to the man in that precise moment and what reaction it might solicit from him. In other words, this is a sentence truncated at the moment the subject's relationship with the Other is evoked – a moment when the subject is interpolated to delineate its own position within the symbolic domain.

The relationship between the detached signifier, its original context, the anticipated signification, and the compensatory hallucination can be better elucidated by referring to Lacan's representation of the retroactive movement of meaning-making (Lacan [1960] 2006, 681–683; Fink 2004, 113–114). Lacan posits that during verbal communication, our thoughts aren't telepathically transferred (Lacan 1970). Thoughts – completed or not – do not travel in any direct way from one mind to another. What is conveyed in speech are bits of sounds, or signifiers. These signifiers are presented in linear succession, one following the other. However, the intended meaning of the sentence – the signified – is only conceived upon the sentence's completion. That is, words presented at the beginning of a sentence only receive their meaning in the context of the whole sentence when the final word of the sentence is uttered.

Consider the sentence, "Look out for your teammates." Prior to the sentence's completion, the word "look" could signify numerous things. In isolation, for instance, it could denote the literal act of looking. With the successive utterance of the word "out", the word "look" could also denote a potential danger: "look out!" However, as demonstrated in this example, it only receives its intended meaning when the word "teammates" is pronounced. At this point, the words "look" and "out" together are interpreted as referring to care.

Fink suggests that this mode of retroactive signification is encapsulated in Lacan's first graph of desire (Fink 2004, 114; Lacan [1960] 2006, 681). In Figure 11.1 showing this, the horizontal arrow in the graph, spanning from S to S' represents the sequential chaining of signifiers in a sentence uttered by a speaker. The process of the sentence's signification is denoted by the arrow branching from the triangle at the base of the graph, symbolising the speaker's intention to convey meaning. Contrary to the linear succession characterising the chain of signifiers, the signification of the sentence is established retroactively. It commences once the sentence is completed – at intersection B – and retroactively endows the words articulated at the sentence's beginning – at intersection A – with their meaning. This is symbolised by the returning arrow.

Figure 11.1 illustrates that in the process of speech production, signifiers are extracted from the Other (the locus of signifiers) and connected in a chain. Concurrently, the anticipation of meaning begins, and the message is expected to arise in one's speech. This message remains suspended until a certain point in the sentence's articulation: the right intersection (B). The right intersection pertains to the moment of punctuation when the intention to speak materialises into signification:

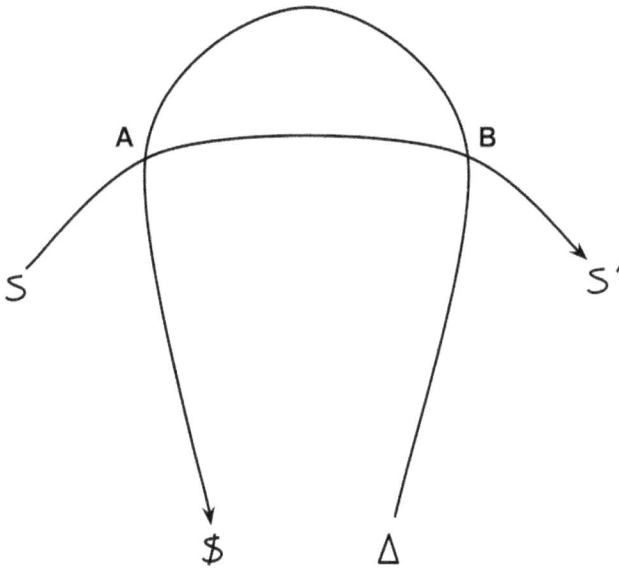

Figure 11.1 Lacan's first graph of desire, demonstrating the retroactive movement of meaning-making and the split of the subject

a message. Thus, we see that punctuation is established only if an adequate number of signifiers have been articulated and contextualised.

Lastly, Figure 11.1 also illustrates that generating meaning induces a subjective effect. This stems from the fact that the sentence's articulation and the meaning it generated never entirely encapsulate the speaker's initial intention prior to uttering it. Language invariably falls short, and the barred subject, the subject under the predication of language, is the precise effect of this shortfall: it is a subject divided between an obscure inherent intention and the signification of what is said. In neurosis, this division is expressed internally: in the split between consciousness and the unconscious. In psychosis, it relates to the disconnection from one's own intentions, perceiving them as originating from the external world – from the Other.

The message phenomenon depicted in Lacan's case study emanates from such a moment of division – occurring when signification is abruptly interrupted mid-sentence. At this juncture, following the utterance of the sentence about the visit to the butcher's, a remnant of the signifying chain is detached from it. The Other, as a repository of signifiers, is then interpolated to provide the signifying material necessary to conclude the sentence. At this stage, a signifier from the Other is imposed on the subject: "sow" (see Figure 11.2). This is a signifier that is metonymically related to the original sentence. But when it intrudes upon the subject, it tends to be inconsistent with the reality of the situation, which explains why the subject is often not reconciled with it. On the contrary, the subject is divided by it, giving rise to a sense of unease.

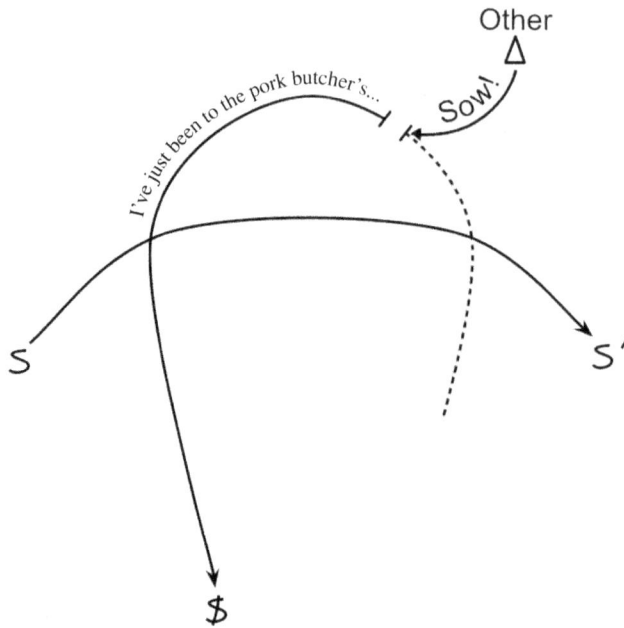

Figure 11.2 Altered version of Lacan's first graph of desire demonstrating the emergence of the signifier "sow" perceived as coming from the Other

Here we observe that the anticipatory suspension of meaning-making remains unresolved for his patient, engendering feelings of enigma and tension within her. The emergence of the signifier "sow" mitigates some of this tension and retroactively seals the suspension of meaning-making that began with the sentence, "I've just been…." It introduces an alternative punctuation to the one that was postponed, thereby engendering meaning. "Sow" will predicate and signify the "I" that was introduced as the subject of the sentence, thus *I=Sow*. However, as the signifier "sow" is perceived as originating from the Other, from an external intention, it leads the woman to the conclusion that she was insulted.

Lacan provides extensive commentary on the complexities surrounding the psychotic subject's relationship with the Other in his seminar on The Psychoses. Specifically, he discusses instances where the subject is compelled to directly confront the symbolic void induced by psychotic foreclosure (Lacan [1955–1956] 1993, 203, 305–306). In Lacan's structural analysis of psychosis, he posits a constitutive psychic mechanism at its origin, which he terms foreclosure (*forclusion*) (p. 321). Lacan contends that psychotic foreclosure significantly influences the structuring of the subject, impacting the coherence of the symbolic order, the subject's mode of access to language, as well as the mediation of *jouissance* in language (pp. 203, 248, 274). Principally, foreclosure eradicates an organising principle from the unconscious that regulates these aspects of the psyche, leaving behind a void that occasionally threatens to bring the subject's psychic life to the brink of collapse. For Schreber, these are life events that put into question his own paternal potency, namely his "virility" or "procreative power" (Schreber 1903, 292–293). In Lacan's case study mentioned above, this instance occurs when the patient encounters a virile man – a man of dubious morals known to be married but engaged in an affair with her neighbour (Lacan [1955–1956] 1993, 48). This confrontation interpolates the patient to a point where her position as a woman relative to men is questioned – a position that can only be accommodated symbolically (Lacan [1958] 2006, 460).

As a result of psychotic foreclosure, the symbolic order fails to equip the subject with organising principles that could define its position in the social bond (Brenner 2020, 86–87). This position pertains to the subject's identity and its relationship with social authority. Consequently, it can be posited that during the encounter with her neighbour, the woman finds herself on the precipice of a symbolic void: a site where the relationship between men and women is left unarticulated, leaving room for fantasies of aggression and bodily fragmentation. This distressing experience abruptly severs the chain of signification, leaving the woman bewildered. The hallucinated signifier "sow" concludes the symbolic suspension as it reveals something about the subject's position relative to the Other when it reappears from within in the guise of an external voice. Given that the man is a disgraceful womaniser, the only possible relation they can have is if she assumes the role of a contemptible sow at his disposal, as the voice suggests. Pertaining to this issue, Lacan provides us with a significant formula: whatever is foreclosed from the symbolic order reappears in the real ([1955–1956] 1993, 13). It is true that the signifier "sow" appears to be detached from the symbolic and reappears from without in the realm of the voice. However, I propose that it is not the signifier "sow" that is the object of psychotic foreclosure. The interpolation to the edge of the void of foreclosure instigates the fragmentation of the signifying chain, which leads to the detachment of signifiers from one's internal monologue. Consequently, these detached signifiers seem to manifest externally, in the form of hallucinations. Therefore, while foreclosure may precipitate hallucination, the signifying elements that surface in hallucinations are not, in themselves, foreclosed.

Lacan's distinctive perspective serves to de-pathologise the psychiatric view of hallucinations (Vanheule 2011, 89). As demonstrated in his clinical example, the hallucinated signifier "sow" is not merely a perceptual disturbance, but rather an attempt to address the state of perplexity provoked by other life circumstances. As Vanheule articulates, "the unchained signifier that comes to the fore in hallucinations sutures the gap that was opened up by the question of subjectivity, thus repairing it" (p. 90). With regard to the treatment of psychotic patients, this implies concentrating on the corrective function of message phenomena. Specifically, their ability to mitigate the experience of destabilisation and, in certain instances, bring about resolution to its localised episodes.

Message phenomena often supply the signifying material that can mitigate the subject's localised destabilisation. However, as is frequently the case, the repair offered by the patient's hallucinated signifier is only partial, and further work is needed to further dissipate the subject's tension. Guided by this concept, Lacan expects psychoanalysts to engage in a dialogue with their hallucinating patients. Instead of probing the patient's departure from reality, they focus on the fundamental difficulty in articulating one's position as a subject, as manifested in the patient's hallucinations. In working with message phenomena, the analyst typically facilitates their exploration, confirming that there exists signifying material capable of terminating the deferred punctuation. This process involves retracing their origin and engaging with their utility in the integration of the subject's world: specifically, their meaning beyond self-reproach and aggression towards others.

Know-How-To-Do with Language

Let us further expound our argument by examining another pivotal characteristic Lacan ascribes to psychotic hallucinations: certainty. In his analysis of Schreber's psychosis, Lacan introduces the notion of certainty. Interestingly, this fundamental component, the very bedrock of Descartes' rationalist philosophy, is associated by Lacan with unshakeable conviction accompanying message phenomena in psychosis. It is crucial to emphasise that this certainty does not pertain to the actual content of the messages. Indeed, message phenomena often manifest as enigmatic, cryptic, and elusive messages. The certainty to which Lacan alludes resides instead in the presumed significance of the message, particularly its relevance to the subject as the intended recipient. Consequently, Lacan describes this as a "second-degree" certainty; that is, not a certainty of signification (first-degree) but a certainty in the "signification of signification" ([1958] 2006, 451). The second-degree certainty in psychosis correlates with Freud's concept of secondary narcissism in 1914.

In his engagement with the case of Schreber, Freud describes psychosis as invoking an "internal catastrophe" and a "profound internal change of the world" (Freud 1911, 68–73). Specifically, Freud hypothesised that psychosis involves the dismantling of libidinal ties with objects in the external world. Consequently, instead of the libido being invested in external objects, the subject regresses to an earlier state of libidinal functioning. A little later, in "On Narcissism", Freud elaborates a psychotic regression from object-libido to ego-libido as a mode of libidinal functioning. This latter mode, defined by Freud as a pathological form of (secondary) narcissism, compensates for the internal catastrophe through an investment in external objects that is mediated by the ego (Freud 1914, 74–76).

This is apparent in paranoid delusions. For instance, in paranoia, the subject is deeply concerned with objects and people in the world, but only insofar as they convey a message pertaining to the subject. Therefore, the radio becomes an essential figure in one's life, but only because, for example, it is perceived as transmitting the secret plans of the CIA specifically aimed at persecuting the subject. This delusion exemplifies the concept of second-degree certainty in psychosis: the radio's broadcast isn't significant because of its content, but because of its undeniable relevance to the subject's life or existence.

Back to Lacan's case study and his examination of message phenomena. The patient confronts an encounter that remains elusive and incomprehensible to her. This encounter can only be comprehensible based on the organising logic of the order of objects shared by subjects in culture – the symbolic order. Therefore, this world of objects, when divorced from any universal organising principle, essentially becomes non-existent from her perspective. The patient, having lost touch with this object-libido-invested world, finds it alien and disconcerting, provoking an examination of her own foreclosure (Brenner 2020, 90–91). The hallucinated signifier "sow" might be said to resolve this terrifying instance of examination of the void by redirecting the message towards the subject's ego, so that the signification now becomes "she is the 'sow'". This pivot towards second-degree certainty effectively dispels the bewilderment and brings closure to the perplexing moment. The ego-libido assumes control, permitting the object to regain its position within the subject's world.

It is crucial to acknowledge that secondary narcissism isn't merely a regressive phenomenon but also serves as an innovative mechanism to offset the loss of libidinal attachments to worldly objects. It transmutes an incomprehensible world into one that not only makes sense but also elucidates something about the subject's place in the world. Secondary narcissism viewed in this light is envisaged as a reinterpretation of the narrative of the world as perceived through the lens of narcissistic psychosis. It creates a tale where every object that acquires central importance in psychic reality does so relative to the main protagonist or the plot surrounding them.

The case of Schreber presents an illustrative example of this process. The messages transmitted through his hallucinations construct a vivid and variegated world, populated by diverse entities and fateful trajectories that concern Schreber. These imagined elements transport Schreber from the precipice of catastrophe to a world imbued with prospective possibilities. Schreber's creativity is not only played out in the outer world, but also on his own persona and body in his transformation into a woman. This metamorphosis is initiated by an agonising erotomania – a form of obsessive and delusional infatuation, where Schreber finds his body to have no boundaries – and concludes with what Schreber refers to as his "*Entmannung*", which translates into English as "emasculation". *Entmannung* is an obsolete medical term that describes the process of the removal of both the male penis and the testicles. The term combines the word "*Mann*" in German, meaning "man", and the prefix "*ent*", which can imply "to undo", "to withdraw", "to remove", but also can indicate the "beginning of something".

Lacan portrays Schreber's distinct form of emasculation as a unique invention; one that assists him in treating the destabilisation instigated by the psychotic process. Lacan argues that the essence of Schreber's emasculation doesn't lie in a desire to become a woman per se, but in his transformation into "the woman that men are missing" (Lacan [1958] 2006, 472). Specifically this is his transformation into *The Woman* (*La Femme*) – the embodiment of feminine universality. Contrary to Freud, Lacan asserts that this endeavour does not spring from Schreber's attempt to disavow his homosexual desire, to alter his sex, gender, or identity, but is motivated by his creative delusions of grandeur, wherein he becomes "God's wife" who will give birth to a new race of man in all certainty (p. 473).

Schreber's transformation thus targets the level of structure, constructing a delusional scene that enables him to be the phallus for the Other (Muller and Richardson 1985, 215–216). This inventive process is distinctive to Schreber's effort to treat the foreclosure of the paternal function (the hallmark of psychosis) by embodying the figure of exception – *The Woman* – and making an appeal to a figure of boundless *jouissance* – God. Lacan dubs this an "elegant solution" as it accurately identifies a site to be treated through its supplementation (Lacan [1958] 2006, 477).

The inventive elegance of Schreber's solutions stems from the instances of perplexity that typify message phenomena. As evident in his memoirs, there's a notable progression in Schreber's ability to conclude these perplexing moments using increasingly complex linguistic constructions. His proficiency in improvisation and utilisation of language to promptly resolve these semantic suspensions enhances over time. It can be asserted that, due to his honed "improvisational" aptitude, Schreber is capable of repetitively establishing the signifying locus of the certainty intrinsic to his message phenomena.

The art of improvisation, in short, *improv*, is a form of live theatre in which the plot, characters, and dialogue of a game, scene, or story are made up in the moment. Often improvisers will take a suggestion from the audience or draw on some other source of inspiration to get started. "New Choice" is one such common improv game, presented in the famous American television show *Whose Line Is It Anyway?* In one of its renditions, the host gets written suggestions from the audience for a place, person, or situation, and places them in a hat. The scene begins when the actors start to improvise a scene based on one of the audience's suggestions. Every so often, the host pulls out a word or phrase from a hat. As soon as this happens, the actors must immediately incorporate this new element into the scene, changing their dialogue and actions accordingly. They must be flexible and ready to change the direction of the scene at a moment's notice, keeping its general context intact.

Message phenomena could be said to situate a psychotic subject in the very same predicament as is the improv-actor in this kind of game. Just like in this game "New Choice", the interruption in the signifying chain signals a break in the contextual build-up of the scene, necessitating its re-articulation. In both cases, the break in the contextual build-up brings about a suspension of meaning that is experienced as an enigma by the subject. In both instances, the playing out of the new context is the acting subject's responsibility. In both cases, an immediate creative act on behalf of the subject puts an end to the moment of anticipation. In the "New Choice" game, the context will be re-defined according to notes pulled out from the hat, for example, "tiger", "wedding", "in-love". In the case of psychosis, the notes all say the same thing: "the ego". The creative improvisation in the case of psychosis always has to do with contextualising the interrupted signifying chain in relation to the ego itself. The better the subject is in this "psychotic *improv*", the quicker the suspension of meaning can be brought to an end.

This brings us full circle to Aristotle's characterisation of the artistic act as the application of form onto matter. As noted earlier, many psychotic subjects demonstrate considerable inventiveness and creativity in their engagement with their hallucinations. Some can even create remarkable artistic productions that are appreciated by others, as exemplified by Jung's *Red Book* (Hogenson 2019). However, in our psychoanalytic engagement with these creations, it is advised that we primarily concentrate on their *form* rather than their *content* (McGowan 2022, 36–37). In this light, the creativity shown by psychotic subjects in the context of message phenomena can be considered as a manipulation of the form of language. Psychotic subjects like Schreber must become adept improvisational actors, spontaneously devising responses to the suspension of meaning in message phenomena: ones that are self-referential. Drawing a parallel with the "New Choice" game, the effectiveness of their improvisations is less a matter of their content and more about their ability to recontextualise and deftly navigate the anticipatory moment, irrespective of the content they interact with. In this regard, they embody the spirit of artists as described in the Aristotelian sense, becoming masters of the *matter* of language by giving it *form*: they sculpt it in their own image. This practice of narcissistic aesthetics bestows their world with a sense of certainty, affirming their position within it, and furnishing a promise of a potential future.

The psychoanalyst, when working with analysands in this manner, strives to nurture this artistic inclination. Drawing on Freud, who posited that the analyst should be well acquainted with literary works, the analyst's role in such instances is to highlight, at specific junctures – particularly where such solutions have a stabilising effect amidst the hallucinatory suspension of meaning – the inherent fluidity and malleability of poetic forms. In such an analysis, the objective is to aid the subject in discovering their own poetic mould. This entails constructing a poetic lexicon, but more importantly, cultivating a unique writing style. Echoing Lacan in his seminar on Joyce, it can be argued that this therapeutic approach with psychotic subjects centres on the formation of the *escabeau* (Lacan [1975–1976] 2016, 145). Directly translated as "stepladder", the *escabeau* represents a small step that allows the subject to ascend to the realm of the Beautiful (*Beau*). The *escabeau* materialises when the subject elevates an element of the ego to the grand ideals of the Good, the True, and the Beautiful. In this vein, "escabeaus … are designed to craft art from the symptom, deriving from the opaque *jouissance* of the symptom" (Miller 2016, 7). They take the problematic *jouissance* inherent in symptoms – those disturbances, interruptions, or pains that we experience in our daily lives – and turn them into works of art. By doing so, they transmute their narcissistic ideals into beauty. Following in the footsteps of Joyce, analysands can accomplish this by refining their distinctive expressive style, which in this context, is the style of improvisational poetry.

References

Aristotle (1999). *Physics*. Oxford: Oxford University Press.

Aristotle (2017). *The Poetics of Aristotle*. CreateSpace Independent Publishing Platform.

Brener, Leon S. (2020). *The Autistic Subject: On the Threshold of Language*. London: Palgrave Macmillan.

Fink, Bruce. (2004). *Lacan to the Letter: Reading Écrits Closely*. Minneapolis, MN: University of Minnesota Press.

Freud, Sigmund. (1911). "Psychoanalytic Notes on an Autobiographical Account of a Case of Paranoia (Dementia Paranoides)". In *The Standard Edition of the Complete Psychological Works of Sigmund Freud*, translated by James Strachey, vol. 12, pp. 1–84. London: Hogarth. 1955.

Freud, Sigmund. (1914). "On Narcissism". In *The Standard Edition of the Complete Psychological Works of Sigmund Freud*, translated by James Strachey, vol. 14, pp. 67–102. London: Hogarth, 1955.

Hogenson, George. (2019). "The Schreber Case and the Origins of the Red Book". In *Jung's Red Book for Our Time: Searching for Soul under Postmodern Conditions*, vol. 3. Asheville, NC: Chiron Publications.

Lacan, Jacques. (1955–1956). "The Psychoses". In *The Seminar of Jacques Lacan, Book III*, translated by Russell Grigg, edited by Jacques-Alain Miller. London: W.W. Norton & Co, 1993.

Lacan, Jacques. (1958). "On a Question Prior to Any Possible Treatment of Psychosis". In *Écrits: The First Complete Edition in English*, edited by Bruce Fink, pp. 445–488. London: W.W. Norton & Co., 2006.

Lacan, Jacques. (1960). "The Subversion of the Subject and the Dialectic of Desire in the Freudian Unconscious". In *Écrits: The First Complete Edition in English*, edited by Bruce Fink, pp. 671–702. London: W.W. Norton & Co., 2006.

Lacan, Jacques. (1970). "Radiophonie". In *Scilicet* 2/3, Paris, Seuil, pp. 55–99. Unofficial translation by Jack W. Stone.

Lacan, Jacques. (1975–1976). *The Sinthome*. In *The Seminar of Jacques Lacan, Book XXIII*, translated by Adrian Price, edited by Jacques-Alain Miller. Cambridge: Polity, 2016.

McGowan, Todd. (2022). *The Racist Fantasy: Unconscious Roots of Hatred*. London: Bloomsbury Publishing.

Merleau-Ponty, Maurice. (1945). *Phenomenology of Perception*. Delhi: Motilal Banarsidass Publishers, 1996.

Merleau-Ponty, Maurice. (1968). *The Visible and the Invisible: Followed by Working Notes*. Evanston, IL: Northwestern University Press.

Miller, J. A. (2016). "The Unconscious and the Speaking Body". In *Proceedings of the Speaking Body, 10th Congress of the World Association of Psychoanalysis*, pp. 1–11.

Muller, John and Richardson, William. (1985). *Lacan and Language: A Reader's Guide to Écrits*. London: International Universities Press.

Schreber, Daniel Paul. (1903). *Memoirs of My Nervous Illness*. New York: New York Review of Books, 2003.

Vanheule, Stijn. (2011). *The Subject of Psychosis: A Lacanian Perspective*. New York: Springer.

World Health Organization. (2022). *ICD-11, International Classification of Diseases* (11th revision). https://icd.who.int/.

Film and Television

A Beautiful Mind. (2001). Film. Directed by Ron Howard.

Whose Line Is It Anyway? (1998–present). Television programme. The CW.

Chapter 12

Judge Schreber

A Neuralgic Point of Social Tensions

Rolf D. Flor

In the annals of psychiatric history, few cases have captured the imagination as vividly as that of Daniel Paul Schreber, a German judge whose personal odyssey through the labyrinth of paranoia was chronicled in his 1903 work, *Memoirs of My Nervous Illness* ([1955] 2000). This extraordinary text not only illuminates Schreber's inner world but also casts a critical light on societal and medical responses to his condition. It was this memoir that caught the attention of Sigmund Freud, inspiring his groundbreaking 1911 case study.

When Leon Brenner (see Chapter 11) and I were invited to delve into Freud's analysis of Schreber, I found myself drawn to the idea of building bridges between Schreber's experiences, as narrated in his memoirs, and the contemporary *psy* land-scape. In our discussions, I proposed that we approach Schreber as an individual who, through his writing, took a deliberate stance – a perspective that warrants careful examination and may offer valuable insights for modern psychoanalytic practice.

As I immersed myself in this exploration, two powerful quotes resonated in my mind, serving as touchstones for my interpretation. Salvador Dali, in his 1930 work, mused that "an activity with a moral tendency could be provoked by the violently paranoid will to systematize confusion" (Dali 1930, 12). Michel Foucault, decades later, remarked, "[i]n place of Lancelot, we have Judge Schreber" (Foucault 1977, 131). These words, I believe, encapsulate the spirit of my reading – a reading that, while undoubtedly personal, invites others to engage with the richness of Schreber's narrative and construct their own understanding of the battle he fought.

In approaching Schreber's text, I do not seek to diminish the reality of his psychosis. Rather, I argue that within the pages of his "Memoirs" lies a purposeful subjective intent – one that reflects thoughtfully and critically upon the very arena of treatment. It is this intent, I contend, that holds profound lessons for contemporary psychoanalysis.

By engaging with Schreber's narrative, we can begin to understand why the contemporary context might currently necessitate a paradigm shift – a move away from perceiving the psychotic individual as a mere object of analysis or treatment, and towards acknowledging them as active participants in dialogue, capable of meaningful interaction with the non-psychotic world, even in the midst of what

DOI: 10.4324/9781032663746-19

Fimiani (2021) terms "extreme states". Schreber's work, in this light, becomes not just a text to be studied, but a voice to be heard and conversed with. The act of listening which Freud always incorporated in his practice is the very foundation upon which we establish ourselves as subjects in relation to one another. In the realm of psychosis and psychoanalysis, adopting an even more dialogical approach to Schreber's "Memoirs" could have paved the way for a therapeutic journey (not even foreseen by Freud), had Schreber, as a psychotically structured subject, ever sought psychoanalytic treatment.

In contemporary discussions of psychosis, there is a pronounced inclination towards normative integration, frequently dominated by psychopharmacology, which often eclipses the individual's subjective narrative. Within this context, Schreber's text emerges as a profound counterpoint, challenging the prevailing psychiatric model with a narrative that defies easy assimilation (Santner 1996; Sass 1995). Despite other shortcomings, Freud's intuition that psychotic symptoms present a subjective effort to survive, along with Lacan's attentive engagement with Schreber, highlight the potential of psychoanalysis to learn significantly by earnestly listening to the subjective narratives of psychotic individuals. A crucial part of this process is carefully listening to how the events in the subject's world may be evoked and addressed by their symptoms (van der Haven et al. 2017). An analyst might have been able to engage Schreber if they understood his acute awareness of the "soul-murdering" extension of science into a nerve-centric psychology, critiquing the neuro-reductionistic approaches of one Professor Dr. Paul Emil Flechsig, Schreber's interlocutor, whose approach formed the foundation of much of today's psychiatry.

To foreshadow the end of this chapter, even though this psychoanalytic counter-reformation is incipiently present in Freud, it makes a significant leap forward through Lacan. Lacan's extension of Freud's general approach, rather than Freud's specific interpretation of Schreber, is pivotal in forming the Lacanian conception of diagnostic categories, a view that could shape a modern psychoanalytic approach to engaging with psychotic disorders (Davoine 2003). This involves a turn away from the dominant drive to diagnose and cure, towards fostering a recognition of the diverse structural manifestations of subjectivity. Lacan's understanding of psychosis, an extension of Freud's general model – which Freud himself actually failed to apply to psychosis, and in that way is superseded by Lacan – does not prevent working with (and even as) a psychotically structured client in a therapeutic way (aimed at decreasing human suffering).

One Schreber, Two Schreber

Daniel Paul Schreber's seminal work *Denkwürdigkeiten eines Nervenkranken* was first published in 1903 (Schreber 1903). It reached English-speaking audiences in 1955 as *Memoirs of My Nervous Illness* (Schreber [1955] 2000).[1] The original German edition garnered substantial attention and eventually provoked extensive commentary, a phenomenon that not only reoccurred but also intensified with its English translation.

During the first four decades of his life, it would have seemed unlikely for Schreber's legacy to be defined by anything like it. Despite facing some personal tragedies, such as his older brother's suicide and his wife's series of miscarriages, Schreber steered his career towards an influential role as a jurist and politician. During his early years in the public sphere, he first gained recognition for his legal acumen and became known for compelling participation in prominent court cases. Later Schreber also achieved significant political success; he was nominated for the German Reichstag at a remarkably young age and served as the *Senatspräsident* of the Superior Court of Saxony.

Later in life, however, due to recurrent periods of mental turmoil, Schreber's professional trajectory faced challenges. The first such period occurred between 1884 and 1885, seemingly triggered by exhaustion following an unsuccessful bid for the Reichstag. This early bout of illness manifested as hypochondriasis, with various physical ailments and intensified worries. Under the supervision of Dr. Paul Flechsig, Schreber's recovery seemed rapid and full, resulting in only a slight impediment to his otherwise upward career progression. Nine years later, in a dramatic turn of events, just a month after ascending to the Supreme Court of Saxony, Schreber found himself having a second breakdown and was admitted into a psychiatric facility, again in the care of Flechsig. In contrast to the first, this episode marked the onset of far more pronounced psychotic symptoms, prompting prolonged institutionalisations from 1894 to 1903 (Schreber composed his *Denkwürdigkeiten* (Memoirs) near the end of this period). His ultimate place in history as an unfortunate psychotic was solidified when, four years after his release, he was readmitted due to a recurrence of symptoms, and remained institutionalised until his death in 1911 in a Leipzig asylum.

Schreber's outstanding early achievements have been thoroughly eclipsed by his subsequent reputation as a paranoid patient with a highly detailed and salacious delusional system. Nevertheless, the reader would be well served to momentarily set aside the more bizarre aspects of Schreber's memoirs and remember that Schreber was from the beginning a person with serious aims. The publication of *Denkwürdigkeiten* was not motivated by a desire for scandalous notoriety, nor to gain sympathy for his condition. To the extent that they even concern his illness, he doesn't depict himself as a casualty of mental illness but rather as an individual with unique experiences who handles them as challenges with resilience.

It would be more accurate to simply say that they were written for presentation to the Saxon judicial system to affirm his right to personal liberty, as demonstrated by the fact that he had the work published with legal addenda and an appendix on the question titled "In what circumstances can a person considered insane be detained in an Asylum against his declared will?" (Schreber [1903] 2000, 313). This purpose, as he himself notes, does not preclude his *Denkwürdigkeiten* from serving the public good, aligning with his life story of civic contributions; something he eagerly hoped for, namely that they would provide insights into other realms of human enterprise such as religion and science (p. 68).

The Noteworthy Experiences of a Nerve-Sick Person

The English title *Memoirs of My Nervous Illness* offers an imperfect translation of *Denkwürdigkeiten eines Nervenkranken*. Contrary to the *tell-all* sound of the English title, the German title guides our focus in ways that line up with serious intentions and should deter us from confusing the text with a confessional autobiography.

In a literary context, the German word *Denkwürdigkeiten* is best rendered in English as *noteworthy events*. Prevalent in eighteenth-century literature, this term often appears in titles of autobiographical accounts which document history-making occurrences to which their author was privy. While the term waned in popularity, giving way to modern alternatives like *Memoiren* or *Autobiographie*, the term Schreber chose for his title is found in the titles of autobiographical works written by important political or historical figures. In German, the term is often associated with things that are not only worth remembering but also offer some form of lesson or insight. By selecting *Denkwürdigkeiten* for the title of his work, Schreber hoped to endow his work with *gravitas*, underscoring his desire for the recounted experiences to stand out beyond his label as a psychotic individual. They were intended to appeal to the courts and the thinking public as "thought-worthy-things" ("*Denk-würdig-keiten*").[2]

The term Schreber used to describe his ailment, *nervenkrank* (nerve-sick) is notably different from the then more commonly used *Geisteskrankheit*, which denotes *mental* or *spiritual illness*. This choice may signal Schreber's attunement to the scientific advances of his time, particularly the rise of neurology as a significant branch of psychiatry towards the end of the nineteenth century. However, his use of *nervenkrank* in tandem with the more dignified *Denkwürdigkeiten* leaves open that this is a strategic reclamation – a redefining of his condition on his own terms.[3]

Lothane suggested as an alternative translation for the title: "Great Thoughts of a Nervous Patient" (1992, 2). An improvement in some ways, but the hitch with this translation is that *nervous* has become a stand-in for the word *anxious*. I think a more faithful rendition might be "Noteworthy Experiences of a Nerve-Sick Person", capturing more closely Schreber's primary aim: not to document his mental illness, nor to merely assert any grandeur, but to delineate his unique experiences and engage with a targeted readership, specifically the nexus of law and medical psychiatry.

It should not be overlooked that evoking nerves in the title introduces an idiosyncratic element, that is, it reveals a personal response from Schreber-the-subject. Why should we believe that? Because it foreshadows a *filum aureum*, namely the opening lines with which he starts the *Denkwürdigkeiten*:

> The human soul is contained in the nerves of the body; about their physical nature I, as a layman, cannot say more than that they are extraordinarily delicate structures—comparable to the finest filaments—and that the total mental life of a human being rests on their excitability by external impressions.
>
> (Schreber [1955] 2000, 19)

He will go on to write extensively about "nerve contact", "nerve language", "God nerves", "female nerves", etc. As Jacques Lacan observed "the terms at the centre of Schreber's delusion consist in an admission of the prime function of nerves" (Lacan [1955–1956] 1993, 26). Schreber's ongoing fascination in the *Denkwürdig-keiten* – a focus on a certain systematising of *nerves* and how they impacted him – is encapsulated succinctly in the inelegant translation *nerve-sickened*.

Even when it is not apparent that he is speaking of nerves, one can suspect that he is. For example, the equally ubiquitous references to *Strahlen* (rays) may not immediately suggest a connection to nerves for modern readers who might associate the term with sunbeams or even X-rays (as they were discovered by Wilhelm Conrad Röntgen in 1895, hence a topic of widespread discussion in Schreber's time). But what may be less well known is that at that time, for German-speaking neurologists, *Strahlen* also referred to pathways in the human brain as identified by Flechsig and other neurologists. For example, *Sehstrahlen* is visual pathways and *Hörstrahlen* is auditory pathways in English. These resonances would have been apparent to Schreber, as we will soon see, because he had been significantly exposed to them by his psychiatrist.

Professor Dr. Flechsig, "Prince of Hell": Neurologist First

The significance of Schreber's initial psychiatrist, the esteemed neurology professor and hospital director Professor Dr. Flechsig, cannot be overstated. From beginning to end, the text makes an appeal to Flechsig as Schreber's interlocutor and antagonist. At the outset of his memoirs, Schreber directly addresses Flechsig with an "Open Letter" (Schreber [1955] 2000, 7–11). This correspondence harks back to their meeting nearly ten years prior in 1894 when Schreber, pursuing medical care, entered the University Hospital in Leipzig and Flechsig, due to Schreber's notable position, personally oversaw his treatment. The regimen included neuroleptics and rest which seemed to provide relief over several months. The Schreber household felt deep gratitude towards Flechsig, evidenced rather theatrically by his wife displaying Flechsig's photograph in their home.

However, Schreber's perspective on Flechsig changed after his second course of illness and several lengthy institutionalisations. He respectfully expresses fault with Flechsig in a letter. He does not complain about the absence of a cure from Flechsig. He does not assign Flechsig blame for his institutionalisation. He *accuses* Flechsig of succumbing to the temptation "of using a patient in your care *as an object for scientific experiments* apart from the real purpose of cure, when by chance matters of the highest scientific interest arose" (p. 9, emphasis in the original).

But what exactly is the grievance about? Again, from the start, Schreber puts his cards on the table:

> Dear Professor, I take the liberty of enclosing a copy of [the *Denkwürdigkeiten*] [because] … your name plays an essential role in the genetic development of

the circumstances in question, in that certain nerves taken from your nervous system became 'tested souls' ... and in this capacity achieved supernatural powers by means of which they have for years exerted a damaging influence on me and still do to this day.

(pp. 7–8)

This is the repeating complaint that runs through the text from beginning to end; Flechsig's *nervous system* is supernaturally having a malign influence on his own nerves. The patently absurd assertion may seem to arise *ex nihilo* from Schreber's disturbed thought process. But is it unmotivated? What can be heard in this complaint?

In contrast with the sentimental photograph cherished by the family, we can set another image.

The year before they met, Flechsig published *Plan des menschlichen Gehirns: auf Grund eigener Untersuchungen entworfen* (1883) which is "A plan of the human brain based on my own investigations". This publication's final artefact was a detailed illustration of the brain pinpointing key functional areas. Picture an immense cerebral chart adorning the walls of Flechsig's consulting room which Schreber will lay eyes on again and again during their encounters. As Flechsig noted in his autobiography (Flechsig 1927, 21), he took great pleasure in using this cerebral chart and brain sections (Flechsig's office also showcased *histological sections* for visitors) to elucidate the nature of his research and the legacy to which he aspired.

He had already laid out these aspirations during his inaugural lecture entitled "On the Physical Foundations of Mental Disorders" in 1882, which coincided with his ascent to the professorship at the University of Leipzig (Flechsig 1882). In this lecture, Flechsig proposed a strategic shift in terminology from *Geisteskrankheit* [illness of the spirit] to *Nervenkrankheit* [illness of the nerves]. With this shift, Flechsig advocated for a new treatment paradigm focused on pharmacological or surgical interventions that directly target the nervous system (Flechsig 1883, 51). With forthright admission in his autobiography (Flechsig 1927, 25), Flechsig acknowledges that he is and always was sceptical of the efficacy of any and all psychological therapies.

Flechsig, the fierce opponent of psychology and advocate for reductionistic neurology, is not very well known today. Ironically, Flechsig's life work has been eclipsed by his connection with Schreber. But it would certainly have been known to Schreber that Flechsig was an *outstanding* and famous German neuroanatomist. Flechsig's groundbreaking work as a neuroanatomist gave him a status in his day like Virchow in cellular pathology and Pasteur in bacteriology. His key contribution was the development of myelinogenetic theory which proposed that the formation of a myelin sheath around nerve fibres plays a crucial role in the maturation of the brain. He was the first to observe that myelination progresses in a sequential pattern across different regions of the brain, suggesting a connection between brain development and functional specialisation (Flechsig 1927). This is still considered a pivotal insight into brain development.

After laying out the myelinogenetic development of the nervous system, Flechsig's subsequent work focused on mapping the brain regions associated with various functions and dysfunctions of the brain. He conducted extensive research on psychiatric illnesses, including schizophrenia and depression, aiming to identify the specific brain regions affected by these conditions. His first assistant was none other than Emil Kraepelin, who established a comprehensive system of psychiatric diagnosis and shared with Flechsig his pessimism about treatment. In that way, through his own research and that of his students, Flechsig helped lay the foundation for a medical psychiatry that advocates a stringently biological approach to psychiatric illnesses. Schreber, it should be noted, became well versed in the perspectives of his treaters, evidenced even in the *Denkwürdigkeiten* by his numerous references to Kraepelin's (1899) "Textbook of Psychiatry". a work that offered an exhaustive examination of psychiatry from a neurocentric point of view.

Souls, Nerves and the Subject's Day in Court

Why does Schreber find so many ways to posit connections between *souls* and *nerves*? Why does Schreber pose so many ways *nerves* become *souls*? Why does Schreber raise the outlandish suggestion that Flechsig was engaged in *soul-murder* ([1955] 2000, 34)? This too is not unmotivated.

As Flechsig approached the peak of his career, stepping into the role of rector of the University of Leipzig, he gave a lengthy and well-attended talk entitled, "Brain and Soul" in which he set forth in the opening words his lifelong position:

> More than ever, I am convinced that the brain as an organ completely *covers* the phenomena of the soul and that we are able to develop the conditions of these with the same sharpness as those of all other natural events that are accessible to our cognition.
>
> (Flechsig 1896, 3; translation mine, original emphasis)

Flechsig's role, as he sees it in his own autobiography, would be in the devaluation of *psyche* in favour of neurological reductionism, and the complete elimination of the notion of *soul* – dare I say *subject* – from psychiatry.[4] This stance by Flechsig, reducing psychological phenomena to neurobiological functions, illustrates what Schreber describes as "soul-murder" – a devaluation of the psyche and dismissal of the soul's significance in psychiatry (Lothane 1992, 2011).

Without some sensitivity to Schreber's challenge to neuro-reductionism, translations of Schreber's text struggle to fully grasp resonances. For example, Schreber uses the term "hingemacht" in one of his colourful and oft-cited expressions "flüchtig hingemachten Männer". "Hingemacht" literally means "made done" but carries a darker implication of being killed when viewed in a more figurative sense. (In German, the past participle of regular verbs is formed by adding "ge" as a prefix and "t" or "en" as a suffix to the stem of the verb. For separable verbs, the "ge" is inserted between the prefix and the stem, hence "hingemacht" implies that the action was directed towards a certain location or that it was completed.) "Flüchtig hingemachten Männer" is usually translated as "fleetingly improvised men", an evocative translation that certainly captures the vaporous nature of such beings when described by Schreber. But the resonances of the words in German would allow for another sense: "Flüchtig" can be used to describe people trying to escape. So altogether it could just as well evoke "fugitive murdered ones" or even "the murdered men on the run". This translation would suggest a sort of violent finality that Schreber feels Flechsig inflicted upon him, turning living souls into mere psychological experiments under the guise of scientific inquiry.

Reduced by Flechsig to an object of treatment, Schreber takes umbrage and uses his pen to reassert the existence of souls. I propose that this is the campaign in which Schreber struggles against Flechsig. This is what positions him as a modern-day Lancelot for the speaking subject – although one could argue he resembles Don Quixote even more in his jousting with windmills, an endeavour that Cervantes already knew inherently possesses a moral inclination.

Schreber intended his writings to persuade the judiciary of his right to liberty, and the courts did ultimately approve his petition to rescind guardianship. Following multiple appeals, the Dresden District Court sanctioned his release from Sonnenstein Asylum in July 1902. The court found that:

> What to the court may appear as delusions has nothing whatever to do with the question of his legal capacity; in any case his illness is not of a kind to make him incapable of judging correctly those matters of social behaviour which in law are 'his affairs,' even if one understands 'affairs' in the broadest sense, that is to say including everything concerning: life, health, freedom, honor, family, fortune.
>
> (Schreber [1955] 2000, 407)

The court elected to refrain from determining whether Schreber's *noteworthy experiences* were merely delusions. They rightly limited their judgment to his capacity to live outside of the confines of an institution and to handle his own affairs, taking no stance on the delusions he articulated. They expressed no opinion on his belief that he heard voices that gave him commands; that these voices were, according to him, divine in origin; that he could perform miracles or that miracles were performed on his body; that he was a central figure in a divine drama that had cosmic significance; that his actions and experiences were all part of God's plan to restore a broken world. The court also made no attempt to interpret the special language which helped him structure his delusions with neologistic or idiosyncratically understood terms that had meanings seemingly only comprehensible within the logic of his belief system. Instead, the court simply concluded that neither these beliefs nor an idiosyncratic use of language precluded a life of dignity with personal liberty.

Fortunately for Schreber, he achieved his liberty. Fortunately for us, the reading of his text did not end with his liberation and so he *was* able to make a lasting contribution, albeit as a visionary figure: Schreber finds a way to face psychological turmoil by confronting Flechsig's neurological reductionism – *soul-murder* – in a language of his own. To hear this, one is required to listen to him.

From Freud to Lacan

Sigmund Freud's (1911) seminal work on Schreber, "Psychoanalytic Notes on an Autobiographical Account of a Case of Paranoia (Dementia Paranoides)" carved the path for psychoanalytic inquiry and gave Schreber his very first psychoanalytic hearing. Yet his analysis was more theoretical than clinical, aimed at integrating psychoanalysis into the medical establishment. Freud postulated that psychosis could emerge from repressed homosexual desires, a theory developed alongside his contemporaries and integrated into his broader libido theory (Ferenczi 1924; Abraham 1927). Despite the now outdated conflation of homosexuality and psychosis (Katan 1949), Freud left a critical door ajar by suggesting, albeit indirectly, that delusions might represent a healing attempt, a reconstruction of a liveable world following a subjective catastrophe, a notion that laid the groundwork for future psychoanalytic exploration (May 2018).

Lacan's engagement with Schreber's *Denkwürdigkeiten* provides a second hearing to the first presented by Freud (Vanheule 2011). Unlike previous works that did not move beyond the "*status quo ante*" (Lacan [1958] 2006, 445), Lacan's approach considered Schreber not just an object of study but a subject to be engaged with. This shift is pivotal, as Lacan's work does not attempt to eliminate psychosis but rather recognise the structure of psychosis, acknowledging the self-preservative and restorative dimensions of Schreber's narrative (Apollon et al. 2002). Herein lies the principal connection between Freud's first efforts and Lacan's much broader expansion of psychoanalysis into the terrain of psychosis.

Schreber's insistence on having a soul and not being reduced to *material nerves* finds a kindred spirit in Lacan who sees the value in working with a suffering subject structured by foreclosure without trying to supplant or explain away the narrative they tell themselves. The recuperative moment in Schreber's writings, often overlooked by others, was acutely perceived by Lacan, who saw both the disruptive and sustaining power in Schreber's narrative. This power challenged the prevailing psychiatric and legal paradigms and enacted a form of self-liberation, resisting normalisation and reduction to a mere case study. But, specifically with regard to Schreber, Lacan owes a special gratitude to his work because Schreber not only exemplified what Lacan believed, he *helped Lacan* make crucial discoveries in his metapsychology.

In his third seminar on "The Psychoses" (Lacan [1955–1956] 1993) and "On a Question Prior to Any Possible Treatment of Psychosis" (Lacan [1958] 2006), Lacan picked up where Freud left off, extending and reframing Freud's insights to propose a radical rethinking of the underlying psychic mechanisms within the subject's relationship to language and the Other. Lacan's notion of *Verwerfung* – or foreclosure – elucidates how the psychotic subject, structured by an ineffable choice, rejects or fails to assimilate a fundamental element of the symbolic order. This leads to symptom manifestation in the real order such as hallucinations or delusions, thus defining the subject in relation to the Other. Note, however, the structure of subjectivity taken up in this way is neither good nor bad, it is simply one of the ordinary variations of subjectivity, as indeed every type of subjectivity entails taking up a stance with regard to the symbolic order. This is what makes Lacan's approach so important for the contemporary clinic.

This helps provide a solidly psychoanalytic understanding of the role Flechsig played for Schreber. The role of an interlocutor or antagonistic figure for the psychotic subject, who lacks the essential paternal signifier (the Name-of-the-Father) in the symbolic order, can be seen to create an imaginary other that serves as a stabilising force in the non-appearance of a symbolic function.

In the Lacanian framework, the psychotic subject is defined by a gap in the symbolic order, particularly the foreclosure (*Verwerfung*) of the Name-of-the-Father. This foreclosure leads to the absence of the signifier that fastens another kind of subject via symbolic identity and gives structure to their relationship with the Other (the symbolic order itself). As a result, the psychotic subject navigates the world without critical symbolic reference points that help organise experiences and interactions for neurotic subjects.

In this context, an interlocutor or antagonistic figure can become an imaginary other for the psychotic subject. This imaginary other acts as a stand-in for the missing symbolic function, providing a sense of coherence that the subject does not obtain from the symbolic order itself. The psychotic subject may give this imaginary other special significance, believing that they can confer meaning and structure to their otherwise fragmented and chaotic experience of reality (Vanheule 2011, 116).

The relationship between the psychotic subject and this imaginary other can vary, depending on the nature of the subject's psychotic structure. Sometimes, the imaginary other may be a persecutory figure, embodying the subject's anxieties and fears while also giving a focal point for their delusions. In other cases, the imaginary other may be more benevolent or idealised, acting as a source of support, guidance, or even a delusional love object.

Regardless of the specific form this relationship takes, the presence of an imaginary other can be seen as the psychotic subject's attempt to make up for the missing symbolic function. By engaging with this imaginary other, the subject can temporarily hold off the devastating effects of some real (the unsymbolisable realm beyond language) which threatens every structure of subjectivity (albeit in different ways).

In conclusion, from a Lacanian perspective, an interlocutor or antagonistic figure can serve as an imaginary other for the psychotic subject, offering a temporary stabilising force in the absence of the vital symbolic function. However, this imaginary solution (like every solution to the human experience) is ultimately inadequate, and the subject remains at risk of being overwhelmed by the real. This does not, however, mean that the psychotic subject cannot be listened to, cannot be engaged by the psychoanalyst.

Working with Psychosis

Lacan's "Return to Freud" marked a critical shift in the psychoanalytic approach to psychosis, particularly through his nuanced study of Schreber's relationship with language and the Other, as depicted in the *Denkwürdigkeiten*. Here Lacan observed how delusional constructs could serve as restorative attempts within the crises endemic to the subject's dealings with the symbolic order. In his formative work in the 1950s, especially in his seminar on psychoses (Lacan [1955–1956] 1993) and his essay "On a Question Prior to Any Possible Treatment of Psychosis" (Lacan [1958] 2006), Lacan delineated the structural peculiarities of psychosis, such as foreclosure, positioning it distinctly from neurosis and perversion with a strong emphasis on the pivotal role of language and the signifier.

Although Lacan later expanded his theoretical framework to include the notion of the *sinthome* in his 23rd seminar *The Sinthome* (Lacan [1975–1976] 2016), his initial engagement with Schreber's narrative continued to inform his approach. He described the *sinthome* as a unique signifier that enables the psychotic subject to stabilise their subjective structure through the integration of the real, the symbolic, and the imaginary. This conceptual evolution not only broadened his psychoanalytic perspective but also reinforced his commitment to valuing the psychotic subject's narrative as a legitimate effort towards self-restitution.

Within the frame of Lacan's later innovations, Schreber's delusions and writings can thus be viewed as a *sinthomatic* endeavour. His narrative not only provides historical insight but also serves as a pivotal guide for our psychoanalytic comprehension of psychosis, showcasing the enduring influence of Lacan's metapsychology (Vanheule 2011). By challenging the reductionist tendencies of traditional neurology and advocating for a dialogical engagement with psychosis, Schreber stands out as a pioneering figure who can partner with Lacan, urging a deeper, participatory inquiry into the unique structures and narratives of psychotic subjects.

In this regard, Freud's insight, developed through Lacan's metapsychology, emphasises a common foundational principle applicable to all subjects, whether neurotic or psychotic: every psychic structure attempts some form of symptomatologic recuperation or restoration, which must be attentively listened for by the analyst. In every clinical encounter, the analyst is attuned to the ways in which individuals strive towards these restorative efforts, thereby underscoring the universal applicability of Lacan's psychoanalytic approach. Schreber's efforts to systematise and thus survive the internal upheavals brought on by his condition, particularly under the oppressive influence of his physician Flechsig, manifest a "violently paranoid will to systematise confusion", as Salvador Dali might describe it. Schreber's relentless pursuit of coherence not only frames Schreber's struggle but also champions his narrative as a beacon for contemporary psychoanalytic practice and understanding because he pointed our jousting poles at neuro-reductionistic approaches.

In contemporary discussions of psychosis, there is a pronounced inclination towards normative integration, frequently dominated by psychopharmacology, which often eclipses the individual's subjective narrative. Within this context, Schreber's text emerges as a profound counterpoint, challenging the prevailing psychiatric model with a narrative that defies easy assimilation. Freud's intuition that psychotic symptoms present a subjective effort to survive, along with Lacan's attentive engagement with Schreber, highlight the potential of psychoanalysis to learn significantly by earnestly listening to the subjective narratives of psychotic individuals. A crucial part of this process is carefully listening to how the events in the subject's world may be evoked and addressed by their symptoms. An analyst might have been able to engage Schreber if they understood his acute awareness of the "soul-murdering" extension of science into a nerve-centric psychology, critiquing the neuro-reductionistic approaches of Flechsig that form the foundation of much of today's psychiatry. This dialogical approach not only enriches psychoanalytic understanding but also empowers individuals experiencing psychosis as active contributors to the exploration of their own psychic landscapes.

Notes

1 All English references are to the 2000 edition from the New York Review of Books. For reasons that become apparent, I usually refer to it as his *Denkwürdigkeiten*. [Editors' remark: to situate the reader in the timeline: Schreber's book appeared on 1 January 1903. Freud's manuscript on Schreber's case was with his publisher when Schreber died in 1911.]
2 This is why I have decided to refer to Schreber's writing throughout as his *Denkwürdigkeiten*.
3 Today, both of these words would be replaced by "psychische Störung" [mental disorder] which is considered less stigmatising than the alternatives.
4 A perspective which for some, including Kraepelin, suggested we remove all mistreatment and punishment from psychiatric care, but it also suggested for him we give serious thought to practising eugenics.

References

Abraham, Karl. (1927). *Selected Papers on Psychoanalysis*. London: Hogarth.
Apollon, Willie, Bergeron Danielle, and Cantin, Lucie (eds) (2002). *After Lacan: Clinical Practice and the Subject of the Unconscious*. New York: State University of New York Press.
Dali, Salvador. (1930). *La Femme Visible*. Paris: Editions Surrealistes.
Davoine, Françoise. (2003). *History Beyond Trauma*. New York: Other Press.
Ferenczi, Sandor. (1924). *Thalassa. Ein Versuch zur Genitaltheorie*. Vienna: Internationaler Psychoanalytischer Verlag.
Fimiani, Bret. (2021). *Psychosis and Extreme States: An Ethic of Treatment*. Toronto: Palgrave Macmillan.
Flechsig, Paul Emil. (1882). *Die körperlichen Grundlagen der Geistesstörungen. Vortrag gehalten beim Antritt des Lehramtes an der Universität Leipzig am 4. März 1882*. Leipzig: Verlag Veit.
Flechsig, Paul Emil. (1883). *Plan des menschlichen Gehirns; auf Grund eigener Untersuchungen entworfen*. Leipzig: Verlag Veit.
Flechsig, Paul Emil. (1896). *Gehirn und Seele*. Leipzig: Verlag Veit.
Flechsig, Paul Emil. (1927). *Meine Mylegonetische Hirnlehre mit Biographischer Einleitung*. Berlin: Springer Verlag.

Foucault, Michel. (1977). *Discipline and Punish: The Birth of the Prison*. New York: Pantheon Books.

Freud, Sigmund. (1911). "Psychoanalytic Notes on an Autobiographical Account of a Case of Paranoia (Dementia Paranoides)". In *The Standard Edition of the Complete Psychological Works of Sigmund Freud*, translated by James Strachey, vol. 12, pp. 1–84. London: Hogarth, 1955.

Katan, Maurits. (1949). "Schreber's Delusion of the End of the World". *Psychoanalytic Quarterly* 18(1), 60–66.

Kraeplin, Emil. (1899). *Psychiatrie. Ein Lehrbuch für Studierende und Ärzte. Sechste, vollständig umgearbeitete Auflage*. Leipzig: Johann Ambrosius Barth.

Lacan, Jacques. (1955–1956). *The Psychoses*. In *The Seminar of Jacques Lacan, Book III*, translated by Russell Grigg, edited by Jacques-Alain Miller. London: W.W. Norton & Co. 1993.

Lacan, Jacques. (1958). "On a Question Prior to Any Possible Treatment of Psychosis." In *Écrits: The First Complete Edition in English*, edited by Bruce Fink, pp. 445–488 London: W.W. Norton & Co., 2006.

Lacan, Jacques. (1975–1976). *The Sinthome*. In *The Seminar of Jacques Lacan, Book XXIII*, translated by Adrian Price, edited by Jacques-Alain Miller. Cambridge: Polity, 2016.

Lothane, Zvi. (1992). *In Defense of Schreber: Soul, Murder, and Psychiatry*. London: Analytic Press.

Lothane, Zvi (2011). "The Teachings of Honorary Professor of Psychiatry Daniel Paul Schreber, J.D. to Psychiatrists and Psychoanalysts, or Damatology's Challenge to Psychiatry and Psychoanalysis". *Psychoanalytic Review* 98(6), 775–815.

May, Ulrike. (2018). *Freud at Work: On the History of Psychoanalytic Theory and Practice, with an Analysis of Freud's Patient Record Books*. London: Taylor & Francis.

Santner, Eric L. (1996). *My Own Private Germany: Daniel Paul Schreber's Secret History of Modernity*. Princeton, NJ: Princeton University Press.

Sass, Louis. (1995). *The Paradoxes of Delusion: Wittgenstein, Schreber, and the Schizophrenic Mind*. Ithaca, NY: Cornell University Press.

Schreber, Daniel Paul. (1903). *Denkwürdigkeiten eines Nervenkranken*. Muenze: Oswald.

Schreber, Daniel Paul. (1955). *Memoirs of My Nervous Illness*, translated by I. M. Hunter. New York: New York Review of Books. 2000.

Van Der Haven, Alexander, Greisiger, Lutz and Schüler, Sebastian. (2017). *Religion und Wahnsinn um 1900: Zwischen Pathologisierung und Selbstermächtigung*. Baden-Baden: Ergon Verlag.

Vanheule, Stijn. (2011). *The Subject of Psychosis: A Lacanian Perspective*. New York: Palgrave.

TO CONCLUDE

*It is not fair to expect
from a single case more
than it can offer*

Freud, Sigmund. (1905). "Fragment of an Analysis
of a Case of Hysteria". In *The Standard Edition
of the Complete Psychological Works of Sigmund Freud*,
translated by James Strachey, vol. 7, pp. 1–122.
London: Hogarth, 1955.

DOI: 10.4324/9781032663746-20

Reading Freud's Case Studies Today

Anne Worthington

The Case Study

My starting point is a reminder to us from Julia Borossa that, "it is impossible to consider the emergence of psychoanalysis as a discipline in its own right and as a clinical practice, without consideration of the distribution and circulation of knowledge" (Borossa 1997, 46).

Freud's knowledge was gleaned from the consulting room, from private conversations with his analysands, from those hysterics who by the mid-nineteenth century were perceived as suffering from an illness. The illness was one whose symptoms, without obvious organic cause, included an array of physical disorders and outlandish displays, exaggerated gestures, overt sexual behaviour or a dramatic refusal of sex. With the publication in 1893 of a collection of individual case histories, *Studies on Hysteria*, Freud and his collaborator in the *Studies*, Josef Breuer, demonstrated that symptoms made sense, that they were the logical outcome of a psychical rather than physical trauma, and that this trauma was related to thwarted libidinal impulses. Furthermore, the cure depended on remembering and constructing a narrative within the context of a relationship with the doctor. It is the publication of these single case studies of hysteria that provides the vehicle for the transmission of these basic tenets of his theory which arguably inaugurates psychoanalysis as a distinct body of knowledge and clinical practice. But why read these case histories today? They have certainly received much attention from psychoanalysts, literary scholars, as well as cultural and political theorists. Perhaps there is something in the very structure of hysteria that calls that knowledge, those fundamental tenets of Freudian theory, into question.

From the very beginning of psychoanalysis, the clinical case study came under suspicion. As most scholars cite, Freud had his own doubts about case studies and he thought they read like short stories and "lack the serious stamp of science" (Freud 1893–1895, 160). The literature of psychoanalysis from all sides and modalities, including practitioners and proponents as well as those who are wholly opposed to the field, expressed some uneasiness about the shortcomings of the clinical case study. First, there is an uneasiness about the *data* itself because it is not *objective*. Some go even so far as to say that they are purely subjective.

DOI: 10.4324/9781032663746-21

Robert Michels, for example, describes clinical case studies as the "crystallisation of [the analyst's] countertransference" (Michels 2000, 373). Second, the analysis of the *data* is also thought to be suspect and seemingly only used to confirm and illustrate the analyst's own ideas (Midgley 2006, 132). Third is the question as to whether it is possible to gain generalisable insight from case studies. These arguments tend with varying degrees of explicitness to call into question psychoanalysis itself, both as a body of knowledge and as a clinical practice.

In *Thinking in Cases*, John Forrester draws our attention to a somewhat different critique, citing Graham Greene in *The Heart of the Matter*. He writes, "[w]hen something became a case it no longer seemed to concern a human being: there was no shame or suffering in a case" (Forrester 2017, 193). There is something about "a case" that changes the individual subject, their history, their singularity into – to quote Foucault's *Discipline and Punish*, "an object for a branch of knowledge and a hold for a branch of power … the individual who has to be trained or corrected, classified, normalised, excluded etc." (1977, 191). This is the antithesis of psychoanalytic clinical work which aims instead at an articulation of the specificity of each individual subject without an imposition of a solution to that individual's suffering, offering a place in which the problems of being human can be addressed.

Forrester continues in *Thinking in Cases* to argue that what we "most find seductive in psychoanalysis" is not so much the bits where the case history backs up the theory but "that each and every erotic life conforms to the model, the exemplar, of the Oedipus story" but what is "most seductive in psychoanalysis is its promise to give an account of the divergences, the detours, the idiosyncrasies of the person's life" (Forrester 2017, 11). He writes that it is the genre of the case history that sustains the desire for "the promise of the entirely revealed life, in its singularity and its distinctiveness" (p. 11).

Freud would have been troubled by the impossibility of fulfilling that promise of conveying the full story. Robert Michels writes:

> In short [although not noticing his own pun], Freud gave us extended reports of three patients he had analysed himself—calling one a 'fragment,' [Dora] a second 'notes,' [the Rat Man] and limiting the third [the Wolf Man] to the unravelling of the patient's infantile neurosis, while telling us that a complete history was 'technically impractical' and 'socially impermissible' and would be unconvincing in any event.
>
> (2000. 357)

Of course, there is another case – that of the young female homosexual girl – that Freud does seem to consider complete, describing it as "a single case … in which it was possible to trace its origin and development in the mind with complete certainty and almost without a gap" (Freud 1920, 145).

The question of the truth, the validity of what can be said in and through a clinical case is pursued in all sorts of ways. There are the follow-up cases in which alternative analyses are published, for example, Mack Brunswick's (1928) work with the Wolf Man, and there are the accounts from those who met or indeed pursued the patient of the published case history. Felix Deutsch (1957) came across Dora in the course of his work and published his views on her personality. More recently, Ines Rieder and Diana Voigt (2020) published a biography of the patient in Freud's female homosexual case that gives a quite different account of what went on in the analysis. Then there are the accounts by patients themselves – some famously about their analyses with Freud, but others also. There are those re-readings of Freud's work where the material is reviewed in support of previous findings and where psychoanalytic theory is developed and re-invigorated. A recent example is Darian Leader's re-reading of the case of Little Hans in which the case is re-formulated in light of other historical material about Hans' upbringing and later life (Leader 2021). But perhaps we could argue that one of the most rigorous re-readers of the case histories was Freud himself. When we read the published case histories, we can see how Freud re-thinks his conclusions in the light of further clinical ex-perience. Every one of his case histories include footnotes added later that refer to other analysands or reference the clinical findings of his colleagues, and, of course, he returns to the case histories in his other writings. Take. for example. "Analysis Terminable and Interminable" (Freud 1937) where he returns to the case of the Wolf Man and to cases on hysteria to reflect – perhaps with a note of pessimism – on the difficulties of psychoanalytic treatment and what underlies them.

But when Freud earlier wrote that his case histories read like short stories, he says in a sentence which is less often quoted the following: "I must console myself with the reflection that the nature of the subject is evidently responsible for this, rather than any preference of my own" (Freud 1893–1895, 160). Perhaps these misgivings about the clinical case study are not so much about science or research methodology but the nature of the subject itself. The subject is not the clinical case or the analysand but psychoanalysis itself. We can't say it all and it is through clini-cal practice, through each individual analysis, and each case study that we research and learn and re-evaluate theory. So, when we read and study Freud's published case histories we should do so critically, listening for what is not said and how what is said might be interpreted.

Reading Freud's Hysterics Today: The Case of Emmy

What can we learn from reading Freud's case studies today? We can see the de-velopment of Freud's ideas from his first analyses of the hysterics and then signal how they were developed by Lacan. Let's take Freud's first published case history, that of Emmy von N. (Freud 1893–1895). At this point, Freud was still using hyp-nosis that should have facilitated suggestion. Freud's method was aimed largely at symptom elimination, at eliciting the stories that lay behind those symptoms and then, through suggestion, eliminating the affective response of these memories. It was Freud's experience with Emmy that obliged him to re-think the relationship between doctor and patient. Emmy wasn't eating and was drinking little water, and suffered with many physical symptoms: various pains, curious tics, and the sudden jarring irruption of words. Every two or three minutes, she broke off from speaking and "contorted her face into an expression of horror and disgust, spreading and crooking her fingers, and exclaiming in a changed voice, charged with anxiety—'Keep still! Don't say anything! Don't touch me!'" (p. 49). These were phrases that she can't help repeating. She had a stammer and what Freud described as "clacking" when she was afraid. Freud discovered that the repeated phrases were linked to two instances of fright in the past, one was not being able to keep still by her daughter's sick bed. Freud wrote that these frights, subsequently associated to a later fright "were eventually linked up with so many traumas, had so much reason for being reproduced in memory, that they perpetually interrupted the patient's speech for no particular cause, in the manner of a meaningless *tic*" (p. 93, original emphasis). Freud's thinking about the temporal relationship between different sets of memories and how they were linked to a traumatic effect later led to the development of the concept of *Nachträglichkeit* – deferred action – whereby a later or even trivial event could serve to reawaken affects associated with earlier memories that were not experienced as traumatic at the time. The notion of deferred action appeared again in Freud's work in the *Project for a Scientific Psychology* (Freud 1895, 356). We see its significance elaborated when we look at the case history of the Wolf Man (Freud 1918).

As with many of his case histories, Freud draws our attention to the question of sexual difference. It is a problem that haunts all his clinical work but particularly his analysis of women. He compares Emmy to a man, attributing her qualities such as intelligence and moral character to men. Emmy's celibacy, her renunciation of her sexual desire indicated to Freud a moral character and intelligence that "were no less than a man's" (Freud 1893–1895, 103). Do we interpret this "no less than a man's" as the statement from the patriarchy? Or is it indicative of his own transference? Or is Freud on to something about the instability of sexed subjectivity? Or is he on to what later becomes characterised as the Lacanian question that structures hysteria, "Am I man or a woman?" about what is the nature of femininity?

We see too Freud's emphasis on the importance and function of the speech of the patient. Freud sought to evoke memories. Under hypnosis he asked Emmy again what had upset her. She gave him the same answer but this time in reversed order. He was listening. Emma was able to link her mantra – "Keep still, don't touch me" – to four separate "frights". Freud noted that while these incidents were separated in time, his patient linked them together in a single sentence, "as if". He wrote: "they were a single episode in four acts" (p. 57). He noted too how she arranged the traumas in groups that began with the word "how" and each trauma was separated by the word "and". He really listened. "These words," the words of Emmy's mantra, "don't touch me, etc.", however, "did in fact represent a protective formula" (p. 57). It was designed to safeguard her against any further such experiences. He tells us he eliminated the mantra by suggestion.

However, Freud was not happy with his methods. While he had not developed his theory of transference, he was very conscious of the importance of his patient's attitude towards him. Emmy, he tells us, was highly suggestible and easily hypnotised but at the same time resistant. She was unable to meet him, he wrote, with any favourable mental attitude (p. 99). If he were unable to come up with a convincing reason to explain her symptom, she would give him bad looks. If he took up an authoritative attitude (and we see how he tried to do this throughout the case) and then asked if she was still afraid, she answered "no—since you insist" (p. 99). Freud seemed to struggle with the fact that the symptoms could be eliminated when she was convinced of their origin but would cling obstinately to them otherwise. Suggestion did not work but he was encouraged by the success of the cathartic method.

Freud was explicit about what he learned from Emmy – the importance of talking, and the analysis of the psyche as opposed to hypnosis and suggestion. In a footnote to Emmy's case added much later in 1924, Freud added, "I am aware that no analyst can read this case history today without a smile of pity" (p. 105, fn.1). I don't agree. There's much to learn from the case notes recorded daily in that case and so much to learn from reading these early case histories and from being able to see what my arithmetic teacher used to call "the workings out".

The Case of Elisabeth

The case of Elisabeth von R. was very helpful to Freud as she couldn't or wouldn't be hypnotised. Freud had, however, decided that he could do without it. Elisabeth suffered from chronic pains in her legs and difficulties with walking and standing. Freud, from the beginning, perceived an erotic dimension to her suffering – he saw in her expression not so much pain but pleasure – as with a voluptuous tickling (p. 137). He again drew attention to sexual difference, in how she had taken the place of a son for her father, how she was herself greatly discontented with being a girl (p. 140). We can also see his attention to her speech, the words she used while linking the physical symptom to a series of painful memories. She recalled that when her father was brought home with a heart attack, she was standing by the door and became rooted to the spot; she spoke of being at her sister's deathbed – where she stood. In associating to the pains she suffered when on a long walk, there was her pain at the contrast between her loneliness and her dying sister's married happiness, and Freud listed more. As she concluded the account of her symptoms, she told Freud that the whole series of episodes in her life had made the fact of "standing alone" (as in "being unmarried") painful to her, and she felt helpless – she could not take a single step forward. Freud wrote, "the patient had looked for a *symbolic* expression of her painful thoughts and that she had found it …" (p. 152, original emphasis).

I will just draw attention to two other aspects of this case. First, there is the importance of an erotic conflict. Elisabeth's suffering was not due to her disappointment or even her bereavements; rather her thought at the moment of her sister's death that she could now marry her brother-in-law was a conflict that engaged "her whole moral being" (p. 157). "She," Freud wrote, "succeeded in sparing herself the painful conviction that she loved her sister's husband by inducing physical pains in herself instead" (p. 157). Second, her symptoms were a solution. She was not a victim of circumstance. He was very sympathetic to her situation and agreed that she was right, that he could not help her with the hardships of her life. But he continued to insist that there was more to her pains than her unhappy lonely frustrating life (pp. 144–145). He wanted his patient to see how she was herself implicated in the construction of her circumstances. We see this again later in the Dora case. As Lacan put it in his commentary on Dora's case:

> [Freud] is faced with the question which is classic in the first stage of treatment: This is all factual, being based on reality and not on my own will. What is to be done about it? To which Freud's reply is 'Look at your own involvement—in the mess you complain of.'
>
> (Lacan [1951] 2006, 179)

The Case of Dora

Freud described his case history of Dora as a continuation of "the dream book" and indeed he was treating Dora in 1900 (writing the case in 1901), the year of the publication of the *Interpretation of Dreams*. Freud did not publish anything apart from a small essay, "On Dreams" and the *Psychopathology of Everyday Life* until 1905 when he published Dora and the "Three Essays on the Theory of Sexuality".

There is something very modern about this tale of sexual politics, something that chimes with the #MeToo movement as the story develops in Freud's text. Dora's father was sleeping with Frau K. and effectively handed Dora over to Herr K. to ensure that Herr K. did not upset the apple cart of his affair with K.'s wife. Dora, in this story, raised no objection for some years, even ignoring her sexual interest in Herr K., but in the crucial scene by the lake, Dora refused to be any longer a passive object in the circle of exchange. When her father handed her over to Freud to be made compliant, Freud again gave his hysteric patient a voice. He believed her, despite adding his own twist. He recognised her father's motives and refused a complicit part in this game, and instead confirmed Dora's perceptions (Freud 1905a).

But Freud was committed to his theory that hysterical symptoms are compromise formations that literally express a conflict, that there is a repressed unacceptable sexual wish that gives rise to the symptom. What could be the cause of Dora's symptoms? Of course, it's Oedipus.

At this point, the Oedipus complex is in its infancy. Freud revived the theory in the mid-1920s. However, at this point, it is a simple set of relations in which the child desires the parent of the opposite sex and feels hostility to and rivalry with the same-sexed parent. It's curious because, despite his contention of a universal bisexual "disposition", Freud can't quite believe it. He worked, again and again, with an assumption of natural, or inevitable heterosexuality. If it's repressed, it has to be brought to consciousness to eradicate the symptom. As a result, in Freud's take on the infamous scene at the lake, he imagined that Dora was aware of Herr K.'s erection when he attempted to embrace her, she was aroused by this but her desire for her father's friend was instantly repressed because her desire for Herr K. was a desire deriving from her infantile love for her father.

But in the "in-between" the lines, a different story is suggested in the margins that Freud added in nearly twenty years later. Dora not only had a repressed infantile love for her father but she also identified with him; she not only felt rivalry with Frau K., her father's lover, but also loved her. Her homosexual love for Frau K. was the deepest unconscious current in her psychic life (p. 120, fn.1). Through the footnotes and digressions, Freud seemed to finally confirm his earlier ideas from the "Three Essays" (1905b) that there is a fluidity of identifications, of aim and object, and a psychic bisexuality that undermines his insistence on Dora's "natural" heterosexuality. It is a text that again opened up the problematics of sexual difference.

In *Studies on Hysteria*, transference was approached by Freud as an obstacle to remembering and yet the point at which the transference to the doctor is triggered is precisely the moment that the repressed material is in danger of becoming conscious (1893–1895, 301-304). By the time of his analysis of Dora (Freud 1905a), Freud defined transference as new editions or facsimiles of the impulses and phantasies that are aroused and made conscious in analysis in which an earlier figure is replaced by the person of the analyst (p. 116). Freud was also challenged by the disruptive aspects of acting out. The way of dealing with the acting out, he advised, was through the handling of the transference. As he put it in "Remembering, Repeating and Working Through":

> The main instrument, however, for curbing the patient's compulsion to repeat and for turning it into a motive for remembering lies in the handling of the transference. We render the compulsion harmless, and indeed useful, by giving it the right to assert itself in a definite field. We admit it into the transference as a playground in which it is allowed to expand in almost complete freedom and in which it is expected to display to us everything in the way of pathogenic instincts that is hidden in the patient's mind.
>
> (Freud 1914, 154)

The Structure of Hysteria

In "Draft K, The Neuroses of Defence", sent on New Year's Day 1896 by Freud to his friend Wilhelm Fleiss, Freud set out his theory of the neuroses which established a baseline for his research: the neuroses are the outcome of repression, the repression of a sexual experience or experiences that were traumatic. The memory of this is repressed and forms a primary symptom and as the struggle ensues in which the repressed idea seeks to return, new symptoms are formed which are those of the illness proper (Freud 1896, 164). For the hysteric, the primordial experience of sexuality is accompanied by revulsion and fright (p. 169). But this is strange for if the hysteric is disgusted and afraid, we might expect her to avoid the other and steer well clear. For Freud, it is a question of "quantity" – of too much, of excess. So while the hysteric strives to return to this primordial experience, she must also run away from it in order to avoid the fright and revulsion. To put it another way, hysteria involves the maintenance of desire – keeping it alive – with a flight from it or sabotaging of enjoyment when it is encountered.

According to Lacan, "the structure of a neurosis is essentially a question" ([1955–1956] 1993, 174). The question that distinguishes hysteria is that it is a question about sex, typically framed as "Am I man or a woman?" "What is a woman?" Or, as Patricia Gherovici reports as being the current question in the clinic of hysteria, the question is "What is my proper sex?" and "Am I bisexual or heterosexual?" (2010, xiv). Or from my own clinic, the question is "Am I gay, or queer, or homosexual?" "What kind of man am I?" This is a question that has been raised in a myriad of guises which has always reflected the Zeitgeist of the era. This return of a question, reiterated, repeated to assume a desired form, itself mirrors something of the hysteric's desire, bound up as it is with the desire of the Other. But of course these simple formulations cannot in themselves lead conclusively to diagnosis. Such questions about how we make sense of the experience of being human, what we do with our bodies and sex, and how we position ourselves in relation to the Other are not easily analysable. Such questions are not solely the preserve of neurotics. In psychosis too, such questions are troublesome.

The neurotic's relation to the Other is predicated on the human infant's "premature" birth. Unlike other creatures, the baby is born totally dependent on the Other and remains so for years. The "hysteric-to-be" needs to understand what it is the Other/mother wants based on the premise that if s/he can give the Other/mother what they want, s/he will survive, and bodily needs/libidinal drives will be relieved. Although what is discovered is that the Other can't provide satisfaction. Total satisfaction is an impossibility. It is the price of moving from being a *to be*, to *being human*, to being a *speaking-being*. Nevertheless, the emerging hysteric will still try elsewhere. Freud theorised this problem of becoming human, of subjectivity, in terms of the Oedipus complex and castration. The hysteric becomes particularly attuned to investigating what it is that the Other wants, while at the same time she sets up another figure who does know what it is that is wanted, and is deemed to have it – a master: albeit not for long. Once that master inevitably fails, can no longer provide an answer, they will be replaced.

The identification with the desire of the Other explains the classical characterisation of the hysteric as seductive. On the other side of the coin, hysterics often raise accusations about being seduced. And while not wanting to be an apologist for sexual assaults and sexual crimes, there is something poignant in the equivocal slogan *#MeToo* that for me is associated with the hysteric's investigation and appropriation of another woman in her researches about sexual difference and the desire of the Other that Lacan elaborates in his commentary on Freud's tale of the Butcher's Witty Wife ([1958] 2006, 522–523). The hysteric's identification with the Other's phallic desire can give the impression to the other party that he has been offered something, that there has been an invitation. But if that offer is taken up, the invitation accepted, there will be almost inevitably, albeit not always immediately, a rejection. As we see from the published case histories, if the offer is accepted by the other and followed through, the hysteric experiences fright and revulsion, as Freud put it in 1896 and in his analysis of Dora provides an example. His explanation of this fright and revulsion rests on Dora's Oedipal interest in her father evidenced by her symptoms (nausea and the nervous cough) associated with her fantasies about her father's impotence. Herr K. is but a stand-in for her father. Her refusal of Herr K.'s advances can thus be interpreted as further research into the other's desire, an exploration of her value to the other and a refusal of objectification. Of course, as Freud recognises in the famous footnote (1905a, 120, fn1), Dora's interest is in another woman, Frau K., and the question of sexual difference. What does Frau K. have that the other desires?

This basic attitude towards the other's desire can also explain the hysteric's social success as one who understands what is wanted, what is required, how to please. So very useful in all spheres of life! The problem lies with the fact that you can't please all of the people all of the time, and it is often the conflicts that arise from this sad fact that bring the hysteric to the analyst for a reconsideration of her ethics.

Hysteria Today

Hysteria has all but been eliminated from psychiatry and psychology and is disappearing into new sorts of diagnoses. It does seem to remain in clinics of "Ear, Nose and Throat" medicine where *globus hystericus* is characterised by a feeling of a lump in the throat and/or difficulties with swallowing. It is associated with anxiety or severe life events without a detectable underlying organic condition, and, of course, it is more frequently found in women. A cursory search of the Ear, Nose and Throat (ENT) literature shows that here too *globus hystericus* is beginning to transmute into different diagnostic terms, into, for example, *globus sensation* or, more succinctly, it is merely referred to as *globus*. Perhaps, not unsurprisingly, it is never reduced to just *hystericus*. But in the diagnostic manuals of psychiatry and psychology that diagnose only by symptoms, hysterics are these days diagnosed as anorexic, depressive, bipolar, borderline and even mistakenly diagnosed with schizophrenia and paranoia.

While hysteria has been cancelled in contemporary psychiatry and psychology, it is a term used to refer to certain mass phenomena. Elaine Showalter (1998) identifies six modern hysterical epidemics. A discreet example is the outbreak of a mysterious illness among teenage girls at high school in Le Roy in upstate New York in 2011–2012 (YouTube 2012). What was striking about this strange illness is how the symptoms are so similar to those teenage women described in *Studies on Hysteria* (Freud 1893–1895) who suffered tics, distortions of speech, and outbursts of mantras similar to those of poor Emmy. The students from Le Roy Junior-Senior High School also suffered from seizures. It was an illness that seemed to be contagious, and it spread rapidly from one young woman to 11 more students, including one young man. Lisa Appignanesi, writing about Charcot's pre-psychoanalytic hysterics, draws our attention to the importance of the new technology of photography in the late nineteenth century that allowed the symptoms of hysteria to be learned, popularising them such that they were taken up and re-enacted in forms of unconscious mimicry (2008, 129–130). The students of Le Roy High School and their families gave interviews on national television and posted their accounts on social media, much of which is still available today. In one video where a young woman describes her suffering and exhibits the uncontrollable nature of her symptoms, there is a possibility for viewers to comment. One person wrote that watching these girls' tics had set their tics off.

The response from parents and families was to appeal to the authorities, the state, and the experts, to call for an answer, for knowledge. Others dismissed the teenagers' obvious suffering as manipulation, as fake, as being difficult. There were theories about the impact of the HPV vaccination, about a pollution cover-up by people in power. The girls' suffering became a vehicle for others to promote their agendas and theories. However, the New York health department did arrive at a diagnosis – that of hysteria – albeit hysteria with two of its new names: conversion disorder and mass psychogenic illness (Gulley 2012). This was a diagnosis that was not acceptable to the teenagers and their parents. The knowledge of the experts was refused. This is perhaps understandable as the diagnosis of a disorder can carry a stigma and it's easier if there is someone or something to blame. Theories continue to abound as to the origins of the illness. We might wonder if there is something about hysteria in particular that has to be evaded.

There is a fictionalised account of these events in a novel, *The Fever* (Abbott 2014). It opens with the teenage protagonist Deenie being given the HPV vaccination, which was prescribed to girls as a protection against the possible *cancerous* effects of future sex. For Deenie, the vaccination was a painful experience that led to a fever. Shortly afterward, she witnessed her friend, Lise, having a seizure in which her "skirt is hitched high" and everyone saw her "undies"! Deenie thought about what she saw: Lise "lying on the floor, her mouth open, tongue lolling, Lise hadn't seemed like a girl at all" (p. 14). It is something of a lurid tale in which the fever of the title is one of eroticism. As a "thriller", it was well received at the time of its publication. The novel seems to indicate there's not much new in the way we think about hysteria. Its themes are those of quests for sexual knowledge, the sexuality of young women, somatic symptoms, identifications, and the sexual intrigues and problems of parents. Doesn't this all resonate with Freud's story of Emmy and perhaps most clearly with that of Dora?

Hystericisation

In his seventeenth seminar, Lacan speaks of "hystericisation" ([1969–1970] 1997, 33) which he defines as 'the structural introduction, under artificial conditions, of the discourse of the hysteric" (p. 33) meaning that in the clinic, the analyst aims to evoke a question from the analysand. The discourse of the hysteric is one that can be said to push the master, demanding that they produce knowledge before the hysteric disproves those theories (Fink 1998, 36). Hysterics – as we see from Freud's case histories as well as from the reports about the events in Le Roy by journalists, or in fictionalised accounts, or from the testimonies of the students themselves – interrogate questions of sexual difference and desire and their symptoms manifest the workings of the unconscious. They specialise in questioning and challenging the master of the status quo.

Reading Freud's case histories today does just that – they hystericise. Freud's hysterics provided him with both the material for the creation of psychoanalysis and, as we have read, the method for the investigation of the unconscious. The publication of his accounts of what his analysands said to him and by showing his "workings-out", as said earlier, questions are evoked and provide a site for his readers to push and challenge the master's knowledge, demonstrating the problematics of his theories. The published case histories do not turn Freud's hysterics into cases "that constitutes an object for a branch of knowledge and a hold for a branch of power" (Foucault 1977, 191); rather they hystericise because to read them encourages us to take our questioning further.

References

Abbott, Megan. (2014). *The Fever*. Boston: Little, Brown & Company.

Appignanesi, Lisa. (2008). *Mad, Bad and Sad: A History of Women and the Mind Doctors from 1800 to the Present*. London: Virago.

Borossa, Julia. (1997). "Case Histories & the Institutionalisation of Psychoanalysis". In *The Presentation of Case Material in Clinical Discourse*, edited by Ivan Ward. London: Freud Museum Publications.

Deutsch, Felix. (1957). "A Footnote to Freud's 'Fragment of an Analysis of a Case of Hysteria'". *Psychoanalytic Quarterly* 26: 159–167.

Fink, Bruce. (1998). "The Master Signifier and the Four Discourses". In *Key Concepts of Lacanian Psychoanalysis*, edited by Dany Nobus, pp. 29–47. London: Rebus Press. 2017.

Forrester, John. (2017). *Thinking in Cases*. Cambridge: Polity.

Foucault, Michel. (1977). *Discipline and Punish*. London: Allen Lane.

Freud, Sigmund. (1893–1895). "Studies on Hysteria". In *The Standard Edition of the Complete Psychological Works of Sigmund Freud*, translated by James Strachey, vol. 2. London: Hogarth, 1955.

Freud, Sigmund. (1895). "Project for a Scientific Psychology". In *The Standard Edition of the Complete Psychological Works of Sigmund Freud*, translated by James Strachey, vol. 1, pp. 295–397. London: Hogarth, 1955.

Freud, Sigmund. (1896). "Draft K, The Neuroses of Defence". In *The Complete Letters of Sigmund Freud to Wilhelm Fliess, 1887–1904*, edited by Jeffrey Masson, pp. 162–169. Cambridge, MA: Belknap Press, 1987.

Freud, Sigmund. (1905a). "Fragment of an Analysis of a Case of Hysteria". In *The Standard Edition of the Complete Psychological Works of Sigmund Freud*, translated by James Strachey, vol. 7, pp. 1–122. London: Hogarth, 1955.

Freud, Sigmund. (1905b). "Three Essays on the Theory of Sexuality". In *The Standard Edition of the Complete Psychological Works of Sigmund Freud*, translated by James Strachey, vol. 7, pp. 130–248. London: Hogarth, 1955.

Freud, Sigmund. (1914). "Remembering, Repeating, and Working Through". In *The Standard Edition of the Complete Psychological Works of Sigmund Freud*, translated by James Strachey, vol. 14. London: Hogarth, 1955.

Freud, Sigmund. (1918). "From the History of an Infantile Neurosis". In *The Standard Edition of the Complete Psychological Works of Sigmund Freud*, translated by James Strachey, vol. 17, pp. 7–122. London: Hogarth, 1955.

Freud, Sigmund. (1920). "Psychogenesis of a Case of Homosexuality in a Woman". In *The Standard Edition of the Complete Psychological Works of Sigmund Freud*, translated by James Strachey, vol. 18. London: Hogarth, 1955.

Freud, Sigmund. (1937). "Analysis Terminable and Interminable". In *The Standard Edition of the Complete Psychological Works of Sigmund Freud*, translated by James Strachey, vol. 23. London: Hogarth, 1955.

Gherovici, Patricia. (2010). *Please Select Your Gender*. New York: Routledge.

Gulley, Neale. (2012) "School's End Clears Up New York Student's Mystery Twitching." Reuters, 22 June. Available at: https://www.reuters.com/article/tech-students-twitcnew-york-h-idINL2E8HME6220120623# (accessed July 2022),

Lacan, Jacques. (1951). "Presentation on Transference". In *Écrits: The First Complete Edition in English*, translated by Bruce Fink, pp. 176–185. New York: Norton, 2006.

Lacan, Jacques. (1955–1956). *The Psychoses*, In *The Seminar of Jacques Lacan, Book III*, translated by Russell Grigg, edited by Jacques-Alain Miller. London: Routledge, 1993.

Lacan, Jacques. (1958). "The Direction of the Treatment and the Principles of Its Power". In *Écrits: The First Complete Edition in English*, translated by Bruce Fink, pp. 489–542. New York: Norton, 2006.

Lacan, Jacques. (1969–1970). *The Other Side of Psychoanalysis*. In *The Seminar of Jacques Lacan, Book XVII*, translated by Russell Grigg, edited by Jacques-Alain Miller. London: W.W. Norton & Co., 1997.

Leader, Darian. (2021). "Rereading Little Hans". *Journal for the Centre for Freudian Analysis and Research, JCFAR.* https://jcfar.org.uk/jcfar-bookshop/digital-editions/rereading-little-hans/.

Mack Brunswick. Ruth. (1928). "A Supplement to Freud's 'History of an Infantile Neurosis'". *International Journal of Psychoanalysis* 9, 439–476.

Michels, Robert. (2000). "The Case History". *Journal of the American Psychoanalytic Association* 48, 355–375.

Midgley, Nick. (2006). "The 'Inseparable Bond Between Cure and Research': Clinical Case Study as a Method of Psychoanalytic Inquiry". *Journal of Child Psychotherapy* 32(2), 122–147.

Rieder, Ines and Voigt, Diana (eds). (2020). *The Story of Sidonie C: Freud's Famous Case of Female Homosexuality*. Budapest: Helena History Publishers.

Showalter, Elaine. (1998). *Hystories: Hysterical Epidemics and Modern Culture*. London: Picador.

YouTube. (2012). "Teens Suffer from Mystery Illness", December 3, 2012. Available at: https://www.youtube.com/watch?v=M-Sg0EM8fFM.

Index

acting out xi, 28–29, 33, 34, 55, 64, 65, 68, 189
Adlerian 64
alienation 107
Analysis of a Phobia in a Five-Year-Old Boy (known as "The case of Little Hans") xii, 75, 77, 79, 80, 82, 184–186
analytic treatment 3, 4, 10, 121, 168, 185
anatomical 45, 53, 58–59
Anna O. – Bertha Pappenheim 14, 54, 55
anti-normative 39
anxiety xi–xiii, 4, 22, 31, 32, 34, 44, 48, 64, 69, 77–85, 100–105, 110–111, 122–123, 125, 128, 129, 136–138, 141, 144, 186, 191
anxiety-hysteria 78–79
anxiety-symptom 80
art, artwork 9, 32, 143, 148, 153, 164, 165
autistic 58
autoerotic 80

Bauer, Ida x, 2–4, 9–10, 12–22, 24–33, 51–54, 59–60, 64, 184–185, 188–189, 191–192; see also Dora; Fragment of an Analysis of a Case of Hysteria
binary 42, 46, 54, 143, 145
bisexual, bisexuality 40, 66, 188–190
body 13–14, 16, 25, 31–32, 45–47, 71, 86, 124, 127, 130–131, 139, 145–146, 148–149, 155–156, 163, 170, 174
Borromean knot(s) 115, 130–131
breast 46, 149

cases (Freud's) mentioned: Addendum: Original Record of the Case: 109; Analysis of a Phobia in a Five-Year-Old Boy xii, 75, 77, 79, 80, 82, 184–186; Fragment of an Analysis of a Case of Hysteria x, 2–4, 9–10, 12–22, 24–33, 51–54, 59–60, 64, 184–185, 188–189, 191–192; Frau Emmy von N 10, 14, 185; Fräulein Anna. O: 14, 54–55; From the History of an Infantile Neurosis xiii, xiv, 2, 4, 119, 121, 123–132, 134–146, 149, 184–186; Notes Upon a Case of Obsessional Neurosis viii, xiii, 97, 109; Psychoanalytic Notes on an Autobiographical Account of a Case of Paranoia (Dementia Paranoides) viii, 2, 149, 151, 162–163, 175; Psychogenesis of a Case of Homosexuality in a Woman vii, 27, 37
case presentation xiii, 2–3
case study, case studies xv–xvii, 1, 4–5, 55–56, 62, 79, 86, 124, 134, 157, 159, 161, 163, 167, 175, 183–185
castration xii–xiii, 30, 53–54, 57–59, 63, 69, 70–71, 78–84, 86, 122, 128, 135–138, 141, 144, 146, 149, 190
castration anxiety xiii, 69, 122, 128, 136, 138, 144
castration complex xii, 53–54, 57, 77, 84
childhood vii, 25, 31, 79, 82, 85–86, 89–91, 94–95, 100, 110, 121–122, 124, 126–128, 138
Csonka, Margaretha vii, xi, 37, 58; see also Psychogenesis of a Case of Homosexuality in a Woman; Young Homosexual Woman
cis, cisgender 40–42
clitoris 69
compulsion(s) 99, 112, 124–125, 141, 189; compulsion to repeat 189; compulsive 34, 112; compulsive act 124; see also repetition compulsion

delusion, delusions xv, 27, 44, 128–129,
    131, 140, 142–143, 162–164, 169, 171,
    174–177
delusional system, delusional construct 44,
    143, 163, 169, 177
demand 20, 26, 29, 33, 59–60, 65, 68, 70,
    101–103, 105, 124, 143, 192; Other's 124
demand for love 33, 60, 70
desire: homosexual 61–63, 164; hysteric's
    x, 30, 53, 190; mother's 20, 54, 59, 83,
    137, 142; (of the) Other 53, 68, 102,
    104, 190; Other's xvi, 53, 116, 131,
    190; other's 191; phallic 190; same sex
    61–63, 164
desire, object cause of (*objet a, objet
    petit a*) 64, 68
diagnosis xiii, 12, 41, 121, 123–124, 128,
    139, 142, 153, 173, 190, 192
discourse: analyst's 29–30; hysteric's
    29–30, 192; Lacanian 40, 44; master's
    29; sex and gender 45–45, 48
displacement 54, 57
Dora (Ida Bauer) x, 2–4, 9–10, 12–22,
    24–33, 51–54, 59–60, 64, 184–185,
    188–189, 191–192; *see also* Fragment
    of an Analysis of a Case of Hysteria
dream, dreams, dreaming xiii, 10, 18–22,
    24, 26, 28, 32–34, 54, 67–68, 78, 111,
    116, 121–125, 127, 129, 132, 134,
    137, 141
drive xi, 61, 71, 103, 105–107, 113–14,
    137–139, 141–142, 148, 168; anal 124,
    137, 139, 140–141; death xi, 71, 114,
    129; life 114; oral 34, 61, 82; partial
    139; scopic, scopophilic 103, 137–138,
    140–142
DSM 109, 153

ego 26–27, 63, 65–67, 80, 113, 127–131,
    162–165
ego ideal 43, 65, 125
Elisabeth von R. (Ilona Weiss) 17, 187
Emmy von N. (Fanny Moser – Baroness)
    10, 14, 185–187, 191–192
enjoyment(s) xii, 19, 22, 30, 34, 80,
    99–102, 104, 106–107, 190; addictive
    22; dangerous 102; excessive 101;
    impossible 34; Other's 102; sexual 19;
    as traumatic 101; unknown 30; *see also*
    jouissance
enunciation 3, 5, 116
erotomania 147, 163
ethics, psychoanalytic ethics 127, 149, 191

fantasy 28, 54, 63–64, 69, 86, 101, 113,
    122, 125, 126–127, 189; fundamental
    16, 18; primal 126–127
father xi, 12, 15–17, 19–20, 24–32, 47,
    50–60, 63–64, 66–70, 77–84, 89–92,
    94–95, 101–102, 105–107, 115–116,
    122, 126, 128, 129, 132, 137–139, 142,
    187–189, 191
father function, function of the father 138–39
feminine 34, 58; attitude 136; failing
    12; homosexuality 62; impulses 138;
    jouissance 30, 99; Oedipus complex 58;
    position(ing) 57, 63, 140; sexuality 57,
    63–64; universality 163
femininity 25, 55, 57–60, 63, 67, 69–71,
    136, 186
fixation 41, 94
Flechsig, Paul Emil 168–169, 171–174,
    176–178
flesh: concept of 155; pleasures of 71; real
    of 71
foreclosure xix, xv, 46, 131, 135–137, 139,
    141, 146, 160–161, 163–164, 175–177
Foucault, Michel 12, 14, 167, 193
Fragment of an Analysis of a Case of
    Hysteria x, 2–4, 9–10, 12–22, 24–33,
    51–54, 59–60, 64, 184–185, 188–189,
    191–192; *see also* Dora
free association viii, xiii, xiv, 2, 4, 121,
    123–132, 134–146, 149, 184–186
Freudian xvii, 27, 39, 41, 54, 68, 92, 101, 109,
    113, 114, 128, 135, 136, 137, 138, 145, 183
Freudian–Lacanian iii, xvii, 69
From the History of an Infantile Neurosis
    vii, xi, 37, 58; *see also* Wolf Man
frustration 32, 41, 58, 60, 67

gaslighting x, 15–16, 22
gaze, scopic 4, 21, 26, 28, 56, 63, 70, 103,
    137–138, 140–143, 149, 158
gender, gender identity xi, 4, 12, 39–48, 56,
    63–65, 164
Graf, Herbert xii, 75, 77, 79, 80, 82,
    184–186; *see also* Analysis of a Phobia
    in a Five-Year-Old Boy; Little Hans

hallucination xiii, xiv, xv, 4, 131–136, 140,
    142, 153–158, 161–163, 165, 176
hate 30, 51, 58, 66, 68, 147
homophobia xi
homosexuality xi, 4, 27–29, 39, 42–43,
    50–51, 53, 55–58, 60–66, 67–71, 175,
    164, 184–185, 189, 190

homosexuality, female 27–29, 39, 53, 55–56, 62, 69–70, 184–185
hysteria, hysterics, hysterical x, xi, xii, xiv, xv, xvi, 2–4, 9–16, 18–20, 24–30, 34, 42, 50–51, 53–54, 61, 69, 77–79, 102, 109–110, 113, 123, 183, 186, 188–189, 190–192
hysteria and trauma 16

identification xvi, 1, 16, 26–27, 43, 45, 51, 54, 56, 61–63, 65–66, 68, 81, 131, 138, 140, 190
imaginary father 59–60, 137
imaginary identification 51, 138, 140, 148
imaginary order, imaginary register 18, 25–28, 56, 59, 68, 81, 91, 115, 117, 127–131, 137–139, 143, 177
imaginary object, imaginary other 33, 54, 81, 176
imaginary phallus 54, 81–83, 149
improv, improvisation xv, 153, 164–165

jealousy 31, 59, 66, 69, 70, 78, 83
jouissance xiii, 18, 22, 30–32, 34, 54, 64–65, 70, 82, 101–106, 130–131, 137, 139, 141–147, 149, 160, 164–165; feminine 30, 99; phallic 30, 65, 69, 84; (as) Other 30; real 139, 142–143, 146, 148; (of the) symptom 165

Lacanian xi, xii, xiv, xvii, 16, 17, 39–43, 48, 81, 99, 115, 134–135, 141–144, 148, 149, 168, 176, 186
lalangue 145, 148
language xv, xvi, 3–4, 33–34, 47, 56, 106, 131, 139, 142–149, 153, 156, 159–160, 162, 164–165, 171, 174–177
Lanzer, Ernst xiii, 109–110, 112, 114, 116; *see also* Addendum: Original Record of the Case; Notes Upon a Case of Obsessional Neurosis; Rat Man
latency phase 69
lesbian, lesbianism 55, 60, 69
libido, libidinal 57, 78–79, 148, 162–163, 175, 183, 190
Little Hans (Herbert Graf) xii, 75, 77, 79, 80, 82, 184–186; *see also* Analysis of a Phobia in a Five-Year-Old Boy
love 9, 12, 14–15, 17–18, 20–22, 25–29, 31, 33, 40, 43, 47, 51–55, 58, 60, 62, 64–67, 69, 70–71, 82–83, 125, 137, 140, 147, 164, 176, 189
love, courtly 17–18, 52
love, demand for 33, 60, 70

mania 111
masculine sexuality, masculinity 19, 25, 33–34, 41, 46–47, 54, 58, 69, 132, 140
message phenomena xiv, xv, 4, 153, 156–59, 161–65
metaphor xii, 28–29, 54, 60, 83–84, 124, 131, 137, 139, 142
metaphor, paternal xii, 83–84, 131, 137, 139, 142, 146, 147, 149; *see also* paternal metaphor
metonymy, metonymic 28–29, 32, 81, 159
mirror image, mirror phase 32, 41, 128, 141
mother 14–15, 26, 28, 31, 33, 44–45, 51, 54, 56–60, 62–63, 66–70, 77–78, 80–86, 89–92, 137–138, 140, 142–143, 149, 157, 190
mourning 63, 65–66, 139
myth xii, 45, 59, 63, 85, 110, 115, 122

Nachträglichkeit 186
Name-of-the-Father 44–45, 64, 83–84, 131–132, 134, 137, 139, 142–146, 149, 176
narcissism 186
negation 126
neologisms 174
neuro-reductionism, neuro-reductionist xv, 4–5, 168, 173, 177–178
neurosis, neurotic xii, xiii, xiv, 2, 4, 10–13, 16, 27–28, 40–44, 50, 54, 77, 81, 89, 92, 99–102, 105, 109–110, 112–114, 116–117, 121, 123–124, 127, 130–132, 135–136, 143–147, 149, 159, 176–177, 189
neurosis, obsessional xii, xiii, xiv, 4, 12, 99–102, 109–110, 112–114, 117, 123–124, 127, 132, 136; *see also* obsessional neurosis
non–binary 40–43
normative, normativity xi, 39–40, 49, 57, 84, 168, 177
Notes Upon a Case of Obsessional Neurosis viii, xiii, 97, 109; *see also* Lanzer, Ernst; Rat Man

object a (*objet a*) 45, 56, 64–65, 68, 115, 125, 137, 139, 146
object choice 39, 40–42, 55, 57–59, 61–64, 140
object relation(s) xii, 27, 40, 35, 74, 77, 81, 88, 95
obsession(n) xii, xiii, 99–106, 109–114, 116, 124, 140, 142; *see also* obsessional neurosis
obsessional (adj) xii, 101, 105; affects 110; analysand 125, 110; behaviors 122;

defences xiii, 125; desire 124–125; ideas 111–112, 116–117; nature 140; states 111; structure 124; symptoms 124, 142; way 105; women 99; world 101; *see also* obsessional neurosis

obsessional (subj), obsessional subjects xii, xxii, 4, 27, 99–106, 115–117, 12, 123–125, 142

obsessional neurosis xii, xiii, xiv, 4, 12, 99–102, 109–110, 112–114, 117, 123–124, 127, 132, 136; *see also* neurosis, obsessional

oedipal viii, xiv, 4, 58, 62, 66, 70, 80, 84, 95, 142, 149, 191; –isation 83; post– 134

Other (big Other) xv, 14, 16, 27, 29, 30, 33, 53, 57, 64, 68, 84, 99, 101–107, 131, 140, 143–149, 158–161, 164, 175–178, 190

Pankejeff, Sergius (Sergei) Konstantinovich xiii, xiv, 2, 4, 119, 121, 123–132, 134–146, 149, 184–186; *see also* From the History of an Infantile Neurosis; Wolf Man

paranoia, paranoiac 26, 44, 48, 62, 110, 123, 129, 131, 141–142, 147–148, 162, 167, 191

passage to the act (*passage à l'acte*) xi, 64–65

paternal metaphor xii, 83–84, 131, 137, 139, 142, 146, 147, 149

penis 18–19, 27, 54, 58–59, 82, 86, 99, 122, 149, 163; child as a symbolic substitute for 58

penis envy 62, 69

perversion, perverse, perversely 2, 11, 28, 44, 109, 135, 177

phallic: criteria 58; desire 190; function 44, 52, 63, 70–71; *jouissance* 65; law 44; sexuality 69, 190; signification 58; value 85

phallus 18, 48, 52–53, 58–60, 63–64, 70, 81–83, 164; child's identification as 81; imaginary 54, 81–83, 149; mother's 81; paternal 59; (as) signifier 53–54; symbolic 53, 59, 81, 116, 149

physical trauma 183

phobia(s), phobic xii, 18–19, 33, 60, 77–85, 89, 91, 93, 95, 109, 123

pleasure(s) 2, 97, 100–101, 110, 172, 187; of the flesh 71

pleasure principle 101

pousse-à-la-femme 45

procrastination xiii, 103, 105

preoedipal, preoedipality 56–58, 61, 81, 84

privation 59, 70, 82

psychiatry 11, 123, 168, 170, 173, 178, 191

Psychoanalytic Notes on an Autobiographical Account of a Case of Paranoia (Dementia Paranoides) (also known as "the case of Schreber") viii, 2, 149, 151, 162–163, 175

Psychogenesis of a Case of Homosexuality in a Woman vii, 27, 37

psychosis, psychotic viii, xiii, xiv, xv, xxi, 4, 11, 26–27, 40, 42–43, 45–46, 68, 109, 124, 127–131, 134–135, 136–150, 153–160, 162, 164–169, 175, 177–178, 190; onset of 131, 169; ordinary psychosis 136, 142, 146–147; triggering of 131, 138–139, 147

psychotic feminization 45

psychotic subject 127, 146–147, 155, 160, 164, 175–177

queer xi, 71, 190; theorists 70; theory iii, 4, 47, 64

Rat Man (Ernst Lanzer) iii, viii, xii, xiii, xxii, 2, 4, 9, 10, 97, 99–107, 109–117; *see also* Notes Upon a Case of Obsessional Neurosis

reaction formation 62, 141

real (Lacanian) 25, 30, 47, 56, 59–60, 64, 71, 115, 128, 130–132, 137–138, 141–144, 146, 148, 161, 176–177; (of the) body 127; foreclosure (of) 146; (of) gender 47; (as) invasive 141–142; (of) *jouissance* 131, 139, 142–143, 146; lack 59; mother 82; mythical 59; (of) separation 105–107; (of the) symptom 105–106; without law 143

real (in reality): castration 54; cause of cure 13; children 92; cure 171; lack 59; life 22; –life material 85; object 54, 82; panic 18; realistic fear 80; trans person 45; woman 41; world 114

reality 26, 34, 46–47, 56, 68, 111, 126, 128, 136–139, 153, 156, 159, 167, 176, 188; (of) castration 136–137; clinical 4, 143; departure from 162; "objective" 153; physical 114; psychic 163; "reality" 127, 129; subjective 156

repetition 115, 116, 132; repetition compulsion 141, 189; repetitive acts 116; *see also* compulsion to repeat

repression 64, 78–79, 106, 110, 136, 144–145, 189

resistance(s) xx, 10, 41, 47, 104, 121, 136

schizophrenia 109, 148, 153–54, 173, 191
Schreber (Judge Daniel Paul Schreber)
iii, viii, xiv, xv, xxii, 2, 4, 26, 142, 151,
153, 155–156, 161–165, 167–178;
see also Psychoanalytic Notes on an
Autobiographical Account of a Case of
Paranoia
Seminar, Lacan's Seminar 0 (Wolfman)
137, 139, 141; Seminar I 25; Seminar
III xiii, 26, 51, 127, 137, 146, 157, 160,
175, 177; Seminar IV xii, 27, 81, 83,
92; Seminar V 16, 20, 51, 53; Seminar
VI 87, 144; Seminar VI xix, 11, 144;
Seminar VII 101; Seminar X 64, 124–
125; Seminar XI 132, 142, 146; Seminar
XVII 29, 192; Seminar XX 64; Seminar
XXIII 130–131, 135, 146, 165, 177
separation 31, 34, 58, 85, 102–104, 107,
110, 149
sexual orientation xi, 63
sexuality iii, xi, xvi, 10, 13–14, 20, 34, 39,
43, 44, 50, 60, 61, 64, 69, 70, 88–89,
94–95, 124, 188–189, 192; bi– 32; boys'
59; (in) childhood 89, 92, 94, 95; female
14–15, 25, 51, 60, 64, 72; feminine 57,
63; genital 50; human 50; infantile 81;
male 19; phallic 69, 190; theories of 61;
trauma of xvi
sexual difference xvi, xx, 33, 54, 56, 63,
137, 186–187, 189–191, 193
sexual trauma 5
sexuation xi, xx, 47–48
signifier(s) 3, 21, 27–28, 30–34, 53–54,
58, 68, 82–6, 92, 106–107, 115–116,
125, 130–131, 137, 139, 145, 147–148,
157–161, 163, 176–177
sinthome x, 4, 16–19, 130–132, 135, 148,
177; symptom (as sinthome) 16
social bond 145, 147–149, 161, 164
speech xvi, 24–26, 29, 33–34, 86, 93, 100,
106, 132, 139, 145, 147–148, 156, 158,
186–187, 191
Studies in Hysteria (Freud) 1, 2, 17, 29
subject i, xv, xix, xx, 3–4, 13–14, 16, 20,
22, 25, 27–30, 41–42, 45–46, 48, 63–66,
68, 80–81, 93, 99, 101, 104, 106–107,
115, 124–125, 127–129, 130–132, 135,
137, 138, 139, 140, 143–149, 154–165,
168, 170, 173–178, 184–185; barred
22, 149, 159; castrated 81; (of the)
enunciation 3; human 84, 99, 106, 146;

hysterical 25; obsessional xii, 99, 102;
psychoanalytic 41; (of) psychosis 135;
stability for 16; truth of 3; speaking
131–132, 174
subject-supposed-to-know 103
suicide(s) xi, 27–28, 50–52, 55–56, 60–61,
63–64, 68, 70, 90–91, 139, 169; suicidal
xi, 28, 33, 61, 64, 70–71; see also
passage to the act
symbolization 129
symptom(s) xi, xii, xiii, 3–4, 11–12, 15–18,
25, 27–28, 31–34, 40, 42, 50, 65, 70,
78–4, 11–12, 15–18, 25, 27, 28, 31–33,
40, 50, 56, 65, 70, 78, 80, 83–84, 87–89,
93–95, 100–107, 111, 117, 123–124,
126–127, 130–131, 135, 140–144, 146–
147, 149, 165, 168, 169, 176, 178, 183,
185, 187–189, 191–193; analyst's vii,
4, 39, 42; –atic 79, 143, 146; –atically
56; –atizing 2; –atologic 177; hysterical
34–35; –metaphor (of neurosis) 131;
psychotic 169

Three Essays on the Theory of Sexuality
188, 193
transference x, xii, xiii, xv, xvi, 2, 3, 23–25,
28–29, 32, 50, 54, 64, 65–68, 71, 101,
105, 107, 109–111, 115–117, 118, 132,
145–147, 150, 186, 189, 194
trans xi, 40–42, 44–45, 47–48, 71; anti–
47–48; transgender xi
transsexual(s), transsexualism 44–45, 48
translation(s) 1, 109, 116, 121, 130, 149,
168, 170, 173
transphobic 48
trauma(s) 3, 16, 17, 123, 183, 186; physical
183; sexual 13; (of) sexuality xvi
traumatic 70, 101–102, 125, 132, 186–189;
childhood as 126; enjoyment as 101;
traumatised xx, 145

Wolf Man (Sergius [Sergei] Konstantinovich
Pankejeff) xiii, xiv, 2, 4, 119, 121,
123–132, 134–146, 149, 184–186;
see also From the History of an Infantile
Neurosis

Young homosexual woman (Margaretha
Csonka) vii, xi, 37, 58; see also
Psychogenesis of a Case of
Homosexuality in a Woman

For Product Safety Concerns and Information please contact our EU
representative GPSR@taylorandfrancis.com
Taylor & Francis Verlag GmbH, Kaufingerstraße 24, 80331 München, Germany

www.ingramcontent.com/pod-product-compliance
Lightning Source LLC
Chambersburg PA
CBHW070326270326
41926CB00017B/3771